The ROYAL
SOCIETY of
MEDICINE
PRESS Limited

Heart
Failure

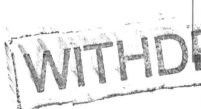

in Practice

Bernard SP Chin

Research Fellow, University Department of Medicine,
City Hospital, Birmingham, UK

Michael K Davies

Consultant Cardiologist, Department of Cardiology,
Selly Oak Hospital, Birmingham, UK

Gregory YH Lip

Consultant Cardiologist and Professor of
Cardiovascular Medicine, University Department of
Medicine, City Hospital, Birmingham, UK

1 Wimpole Street, London W1G 0AE, UK
207 E Westminster Road, Lake Forest, IL 60045, USA
http://www.rsm.ac.uk

British Library Cataloguing in Publication Data
A catalogue record for this book is available from the British Library

ISBN 1-85315-487-3
ISSN 1473-6845

Typeset by Phoenix Photosetting, Chatham, Kent
Printed in Great Britain by Latimer Trend & Company Ltd, Plymouth

Bernard Chin MRCP is a Research Fellow in Cardiology at the Haemostasis, Thrombosis and Vascular Biology Unit, University Department of Medicine, City Hospital, Birmingham. His research interests relate to mechanisms of thrombogenesis in heart failure.

Michael Davies MD FRCP is a Consultant in Cardiology at the University Hospital Birmingam, Selly Oak. His research interests are in the epidemiology of heart failure and the neurohormonal adaptations in heart failure.

Gregory YH Lip MD FRCP (Lond Edin Glasg) DFM FESC FACC is Professor of Cardiovascular Medicine and Director of the Haemostasis, Thrombosis and Vascular Biology Unit, University Department of Medicine, City Hospital, Birmingham. His research interests range from clinical (atrial fibrillation, hypertension, heart failure, ethnicity and vascular disease, etc) to the laboratory (thrombogenesis, atherogenesis and vascular biology in cardiovascular disease and stroke).

Preface

Heart failure is a condition with a poor prognosis, and it is becoming increasingly more common. Substantial advances have been made in the management of heart failure, and there is the need for practical and up-to-date summaries on how to approach heart failure in practice.

This book aims to provide a concise overview on heart failure. We have deliberately avoided numerous references in the text but have provided a 'Further Reading' list, which we hope will be useful for those seeking more detailed information. Management in everyday practice has been emphasized and we hope the book would be useful to medical, paramedical and nursing colleagues.

We thank our many patients and colleagues who have encouraged and advised us on what was needed to communicate the many messages on the management of heart failure.

Bernard SP Chin
Michael K Davies
Gregory YH Lip
July 2001

Contents

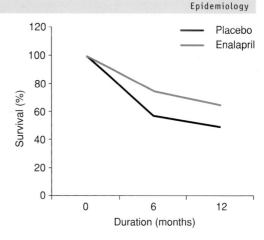

1. Introduction

Epidemiology
Prognosis
Economic costs

Figure 1.1
Mortality reduction in chronic heart failure with ACE inhibitors: the CONSENSUS study. Adapted from The CONSENSUS Trial Study Group. *N Engl J Med* 1987; **316**: 1429.

Heart failure presents a frequent challenge to the hospital physician, general practitioner and cardiologist. In addition, it is fast becoming an important economic issue to the hospital manager and the National Health Service.

Despite recent advances in the fields of cardiovascular medicine, heart failure remains a chronic illness of appalling morbidity and mortality. Severe heart failure has a prognosis worse than that of cancer. In Britain over 200,000 hospital admissions annually (5% of all adult medical admissions) are due to heart failure. Each year, more patients are identified with heart failure. Present treatment is aimed at halting progression of disease, symptom relief and improvement in outcome. Heart failure is difficult to diagnose, however, and many of its symptoms are nonspecific while its signs may be absent in the early stages.

Modern inventions like echocardiography, cardiac catheterization and nuclear scanning have greatly aided the diagnosis of heart failure. Indeed, our understanding, investigations and management of heart failure have come a long way since William Harvey first described the circulation in the 17th century. Yet blood letting and leeches were still in use until quite recently, and thiazide diuretics were introduced only in the 20th century.

The CONSENSUS study, published in 1987, proved to be a landmark trial that showed for the first time a reduction in mortality in heart failure with medical treatment (Figure 1.1). Many more clinical trials have now been reported, and still more are currently under way to find new treatments and strategies that have the potential to improve quality of life, reduce hospitalizations and decrease mortality in heart failure.

> Severe heart failure still has a prognosis that is worse than that of cancer

Epidemiology

Most of the epidemiological data on heart failure were first derived from the Framingham Heart Study based in the United States. The study began in 1948 and has now been extended to include the original participants' offspring. More contemporary surveys such as the Hillingdon study (North London), the ECHOES (West Midlands) and the North Glasgow MONICA studies have helped to define the epidemiological picture of heart failure in Britain.

It is important to note that all these studies used different diagnostic criteria to define heart failure and left ventricular dysfunction. The Glasgow study, for example, used an ejection fraction of 30% as their criterion, whereas most other epidemiological surveys have used levels of 40–45%.

This lack of universal agreement on the definition and diagnosis of heart failure is a major problem and has prompted the European Society of Cardiology (ESC) to set up a Task Force on Heart Failure, which has now issued guidelines for diagnosing heart failure. These essentially state that for a diagnosis of heart failure, both typical symptoms and objective evidence of cardiac dysfunction (such as shortness of breath, fatigue and ankle swelling) must be present. Echocardiography is the most practical way of assessing cardiac function, and this investigation has been used in more recent studies. Where symptoms are reversible on appropriate treatment, a diagnosis of heart failure is more likely.

Much of the epidemiology of heart failure has been based on white Caucasian populations. There is some evidence, however, that heart failure in different ethnic groups may have different underlying aetiological factors and prognostic implications. In the United States, for example, African-American men have a 33% greater risk of being hospitalized for heart failure than have white Caucasians, while this increased risk was 50% for black women. Mortality from heart failure in the over-65 age group is 2.5 times higher in black people than in white people. In a survey of heart failure among acute medical admissions to a city centre teaching hospital in Birmingham, England, the commonest underlying aetiological factors were coronary heart disease in white patients, hypertension in black Afro-Caribbean patients, and coronary heart disease and diabetes in Indo-Asians (Table 1.1).

Incidence of heart failure

Annually, between one and five new cases of heart failure per 1000 population (0.15–0.5%) are diagnosed in the UK. The incidence doubles for every decade of life after the age of 45 and reaches 3% in those aged 85–94 years.

The incidence of heart failure is higher in Afro-Caribbeans than Caucasians. The rising incidence may be due to an ageing population. Significant advances in the treatment of acute myocardial infarction have also led to more patients surviving a heart attack but being left with impaired myocardial function.

> The incidence of heart failure doubles for every decade of life after the age of 45

Table 1.1
Proportion of co-morbid factors in Caucasian, Afro-Caribbean and Asian patients admitted with heart failure to a teaching hospital in Birmingham, UK

Presentation	Percentage	Associated past medical history	Percentage
Pulmonary oedema	52	Ischaemic heart disease	54
Congestive cardiac failure (with fluid overload)	32	Hypertension	34
Myocardial infarction and heart failure	9	Valve disease	12
Associated atrial fibrillation	29	Previous stroke	10
		Diabetes mellitus	19
		Peripheral vascular disease	13
		Cardiomyopathy	1

Adapted from Lip G, Zarifis J, Beevers DG. *Int J Clin Pract* 1997; **51**: 223–7.

Prevalence of heart failure

The prevalence of heart failure in epidemiological surveys ranges from 3 to 20 per 1000 population. The Framingham study reported similar age-adjusted rates for men and women but showed a dramatic increase in prevalence with advancing age. In patients aged 65 years and over, this figure exceeds 100 per 1000 (Table 1.2).

The North Glasgow MONICA study suggests that at least an equal percentage of the population have asymptomatic cardiac dysfunction, with a prevalence of significantly impaired left ventricular contraction in subjects aged 25 to 74 of 2.9% (Figure 1.2).

In the Echocardiographic Heart of England Screening study, of 3960 (63%) participants from 16 randomly selected general practices aged 45 years and older, the prevalence of left ventricular systolic dysfunction (defined as ejection fraction <40%) was 1.8%, half of whom had no symptoms. Borderline left ventricular function (ejection fraction 40–50%) was seen in 139 patients (3.5%). Definite heart failure was seen in 2.3%, and was associated with an ejection fraction <40% in 41% of patients, atrial fibrillation in 33%, and valve disease in 26% (Table 1.3).

Prognosis

Heart failure carries an appalling prognosis. Several landmark heart failure mortality trials

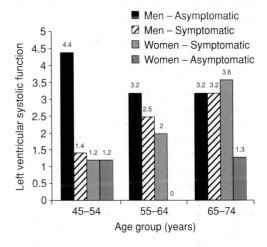

Figure 1.2
Symptomatic and asymptomatic left ventricular systolic dysfunction in an urban population. Adapted from McDonagh TA, Morrison CE, Lawrence A *et al. Lancet* 1997; **350**: 829–33.

have estimated the overall one-year mortality to be 20–30% for mild to moderate heart failure and over 50% for severe heart failure (Table 1.4). In these patients, the survival rates are poorer than are those of many of the major malignancies in the early stages (Figure 1.3). These observations referred to patients with systolic dysfunction, however, and were performed before the days of angiotensin converting enzyme inhibitor (ACE-I) therapy. The use of ACE inhibitors has been associated

---

Table 1.2
Prevalence and incidence of heart failure based on the Framingham Heart Study

| | Age (years) | | |
	50–59	80–89	All ages
Prevalence of heart failure (per 1000 population)			
Men	8	68	7.4
Women	8	79	7.7
Annual incidence of heart failure (per 1000 population)			
Men	3	27	2.3
Women	2	22	1.4

Adapted from Ho KK, Pinsky JL, Kannel WB, Levy D. *J Am Coll Cardiol* 1993; **22**: 6–13A.

Table 1.3

Results of the Echocardiographic Heart of England Screening study

(a) Definite heart failure, by age and sex

	Male	Female	Total
Age (years)			
45–54	2/633 (0.3%)	0/681	2/1314 (0.2%)
55–64	17/623 (2.7%)	5/571 (0.9%)	22/1194 (1.8%)
65–74	20/480 (4.2%)	8/472 (1.7%)	28/952 (2.9%)
75–84	15/205 (7.3%)	15/229 (6.6%)	30/434 (6.9%)
>85	5/23 (21.7%)	5/43 (11.6%)	10/66 (15.2%)
Total	59/1964 (3.0%)	33/1996 (1.7%)	92/3960 (2.3%)

(b) Rates of definite, probable and total heart failure

	Sinus rhythm with no valve disease	Atrial fibrillation	Valve disease	Atrial fibrillation and valve disease	Total
Definite heart failure					
EF <40%	30 (0.8%)	3 (0.1%)	5 (0.1%)	0	38 (1%)
EF 40–50%		8 (0.2%)	2 (0.1%)	2 (0.1%)	12 (0.3%)
EF >50%		22 (0.6%)	17 (0.4%)	3 (0.1%)	42 (1.1%)
Prevalence of definite heart failure	..	..	..	..	92 (2.3%)
Probable heart failure					
NYHA class II or more plus EF 40–50% alone					23 (0.6%)
Symptom-free, EF <40%, on treatment, previously symptomatic					9 (0.3%)
Prevalence of probable heart failure					32 (0.8%)
Prevalence of definite and probable heart failure					124 (3.1%)

Numbers are proportion of screened population (n=3960). EF = ejection fraction.

Reproduced with permission from Davies MK, Hobbs FDR, Davis RC et al. *Lancet* 2001; **358**: 439–44.

Table 1.4

Landmark heart failure mortality trials

Trial	Patients' characteristics	IHD (%)	Treatment	Cardiovascular mortality		Follow-up (years)
				Treatment (%)	Placebo (%)	
CONSENSUS	NYHA IV (cardiomegaly)	73	Enalapril	38	54	1
SOLVD-P	Asymptomatic (EF <35%)	83	Enalapril	13	14	4
SOLVD-T	Symptomatic (EF <35%)	71	Enalapril	31	36	4

EF = ejection fraction; IHD = ischaemic heart disease.

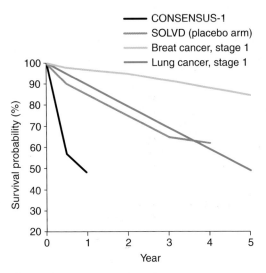

Figure 1.3
Survival probability of severe heart failure (CONSENSUS) and mild heart failure (SOLVD) compared with common cancers.

with a dramatic reduction in mortality, as has been shown in all major ACE-I trials.

Nevertheless, patients with symptomatic heart failure generally carry a poor prognosis. The prognosis for patients with congestive heart failure is also dependent on age and sex, with a poorer prognosis in male patients. Other predictors of poor outcome include raised plasma noradrenaline and natriuretic peptide levels, reduced sodium concentration, reduced oxygen uptake at maximal exercise, and associated diabetes mellitus.

Economic costs

Heart failure now accounts for 5% of all adult medical hospitalization in the UK, with similar rates reported in Sweden, the Netherlands and the United States. This figure has effectively doubled in the past 10–15 years despite advances in treatment.

With an increasingly elderly population, the prevalence of heart failure could increase by as much as 70% by the year 2010. Hospital readmissions and general practice consultations are also higher in patients with heart failure compared to healthy patients. In elderly patients, readmission rates within three to six months of the initial hospital discharge range from 29 to 47%. Length of stay is generally longer (about 11 days) and in-patient mortality is high (up to 30%).

Heart failure currently accounts for 1–2% of total spending on health care in Europe and

Table 1.5
The economic cost of heart failure to the National Health Service in the United Kingdom and other major western countries

Cost of heart failure in major western countries	Total cost	Percentage of national health costs
USA 1989	$9bn	1.5
United Kingdom 1990–1991	£360m	1.6
France 1990	FF 11.4bn	1.9
Sweden 1996	SEK 2.6m	2.0

UK NHS expenditure for heart failure: cost breakdown	Total cost (£m)	Percentage of total heart failure cost
General practice visits	8.3	2.5
Referrals to hospital from general practice	8.2	2.4
Other outpatient attendances	31.8	9.4
In-patient stay	213.8	63.5
Diagnostic tests	45.6	13.5
Drugs	22.1	6.6
Surgery	7.2	2.1

Adapted from McMurray J, Hart W, Rhodes G. *Br J Med Econ* 1993; **6**: 99–110.

in the United States. In the United Kingdom in 1991, £360m alone was spent on heart failure, mostly attributed to hospital admissions (Table 1.5). Prompt diagnosis and treatment of patients can reduce overall costs. For example, starting patients on ACE-I therapy can cut the overall cost of treatment by reduction of hospital admissions, despite increased drug expenditure and improved long-term survival.

> Heart failure accounts for 1–2% of spending on health care

Further reading

Cowie MR, Mosterd A, Wood DA *et al*. The epidemiology of heart failure. *Eur Heart J* 1997; **18**: 208–25.

Cowie MR, Wood DA, Coats AJS *et al*. Incidence and aetiology of heart failure: a population-based study. *Eur Heart J* 1999; **20**: 421–8.

Davies MK, Hobbs FDR, Davis RC *et al*. Prevalence of left ventricular systolic dysfunction and heart failure in the Echocardiographic Heart of England Screening study: a population based study. *Lancet* 2001; **358**: 439–44.

Gradman A, Deedwania P, Cody R *et al*. Predictors of total mortality and sudden death in mild to moderate heart failure. *J Am Coll Cardiol* 1989; **14**: 564–70.

Ho KK, Pinsky JL, Kannel WB, Levy D. The epidemiology of heart failure: the Framingham Study. *J Am Coll Cardiol* 1993; **22**: 6–13A.

2. Aetiology of heart failure

Coronary artery disease
Hypertension
Diabetes and lipids
Cardiomyopathies
Valvular disease
Arrhythmias
Alcohol and drugs
Other causes

The causes of heart failure vary in their importance and prevalence from country to country. In western and other developed countries coronary artery disease and hypertension are common causes of heart failure, while valvular heart disease and nutritional cardiac disease are more important in the developing world (Table 2.1).

Coronary artery disease

Observational data have shown a shift from hypertension to coronary heart disease as the commonest cause of heart failure in western countries in the last 50 years. Coronary artery disease now accounts for almost 75% of all cases of heart failure in the west. It has not been easy to establish whether hypertension is the primary cause of heart failure or whether there is also underlying coronary artery disease. Coronary artery disease and hypertension (either alone or in combination) were causes of heart failure in over 90% of cases in the Framingham study.

Risk factors for coronary artery disease, such as smoking and diabetes mellitus, also predispose to the development of heart failure. In fact,

Table 2.1
Causes of heart failure

- Coronary artery disease
- Myocardial infarction
- Ischaemia
- Hypertension
- Cardiomyopathy
  - Dilated (congestive)
  - Hypertrophic/obstructive
  - Restrictive: for example, amyloidosis, sarcoidosis, haemochromatosis
  - Obliterative
- Valvular and congenital heart disease
  - Mitral valve disease
  - Aortic valve disease
  - Atrial septal defect, ventricular septal defect
- Arrhythmias
  - Tachycardia
  - Bradycardia (complete heart block, the sick sinus syndrome)
- Loss of atrial transport: for example, atrial fibrillation
  - Drugs
  - Alcohol
  - Cardiac depressant drugs (beta blockers, calcium antagonists)
- 'High output' failure
  - Anaemia, thyrotoxicosis, arteriovenous fistulae, Paget's disease
- Pericardial disease
  - Constrictive pericarditis
  - Pericardial effusion
- Primary right heart failure
  - Pulmonary hypertension – for example, pulmonary embolism, cor pulmonale
  - Tricuspid incompetence

smoking is a strong risk factor for the development of heart failure in men, although the findings in women are less consistent.

> Smoking is a strong risk factor for the development of heart failure in men

Myocardial infarction causes impairment of contractility and dilatation of the affected segment (Figure 2.1). Acute heart failure peri-infarction may be secondary to acute ventricular septal defect or acute mitral regurgitation. Catecholamines are initially

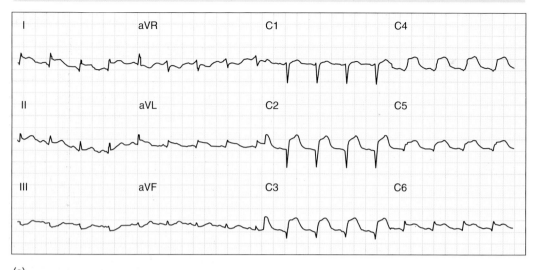

(a)

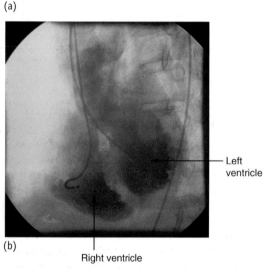

(b)

Left ventricle

Right ventricle

Figure 2.1
(a) Twelve-lead ECG of a 50-year-old man with acute anterior myocardial infarction. (b) Ventricular septal defect following acute myocardial infarction.

elevated in myocardial infarction to provide adequate circulatory support, but may result in larger infarcts and/or arrhythmias while persistent elevation leads to worsening heart failure. As improvements in the management of myocardial infarction lead to more infarct survivors, more patients with damaged ventricles are likely to contribute to the increasing incidence of heart failure.

Hypertension

Hypertension causes heart failure via several pathological mechanisms, including left ventricular hypertrophy. The myocardium initially undergoes hypertrophy to increase systolic stress in order to overcome systemic blood pressure (Figure 2.2). The hypertrophied chamber is stiffer and fails to relax sufficiently in diastole to allow for adequate filling (diastolic dysfunction). Eventually, persistent cardiac remodelling also causes dilatation and contractile impairment (systolic dysfunction). Hypertension also increases the risk of myocardial infarction and predisposes to both atrial and ventricular arrhythmias.

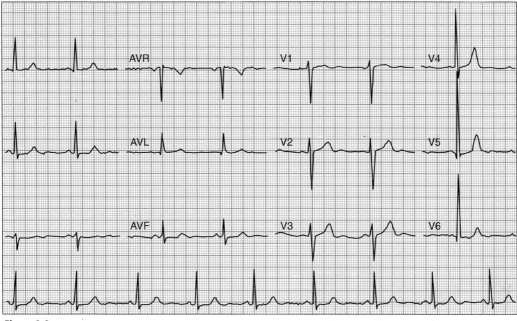

Figure 2.2
Twelve-lead ECG of a 70-year-old man with evidence of left ventricular hypertrophy.

> Hypertension is a risk factor for myocardial infarction

The importance of hypertension as a cause of heart failure has been declining in the Framingham cohort since the 1950s. Recent studies reliably assessing aetiological factors have recorded hypertension to be the cause of heart failure in about 10–20% of cases, compared with over 70% in the Framingham study. This decline could be due to effective blood pressure reduction and control with antihypertensive drugs. This treatment could have further contributed to a fall in the age-standardized incidence of heart failure by up to 50%. Nevertheless, hypertension remains an important and common cause of heart failure in women and among Afro-Caribbeans.

> With the increasing use of antihypertensive drugs, hypertension is of diminishing importance in the aetiology of heart failure

Diabetes and lipids

Diabetes increases the risk of developing heart failure four-fold, and also predicts higher mortality and more frequent hospital admissions. This risk persists even after exclusion of patients with coronary disease, suggesting a non-ischaemic aetiology. The underlying process of diabetes-induced cardiomyopathy is still not known. The severity of ventricular dysfunction in diabetes mellitus appears to be related to the degree of metabolic control. Myocardial interstitial fibrosis and wall thickening of small arterioles have been found. In the Framingham study, diabetes and left ventricular hypertrophy were the most significant risk predictors of the development of heart failure.

Body weight and a high ratio of total cholesterol concentration to high-density lipoprotein cholesterol (HDL-C) concentration are also independent risk factors for heart failure. These factors probably increase the risk of heart failure through their adverse effects on coronary artery disease.

Cardiomyopathies

Cardiomyopathies are rare primary diseases of heart muscle that are not due to coronary disease or hypertension, or to congenital, valvular or pericardial disease. They are normally categorized according to their functional anatomy (dilated or congestive, hypertrophic, restrictive and obliterative). Hence, dilated cardiomyopathies exhibit progressive ventricular dilatation resulting in poor contractility, while hypertrophic cardiomyopathies are characterized by thickened and poorly compliant left ventricular walls that impair ventricular filling. Restrictive and obliterative cardiomyopathies present as stiff and poorly compliant ventricles that fail to relax adequately in diastole for sufficient ventricular filling. The development of heart failure in patients with hypertrophic or restrictive cardiomyopathy is likely to indicate an advanced or end-stage disease state.

Dilated cardiomyopathies are more common than hypertrophic and restrictive cardiomyopathies. Obliterative cardiomyopathy is essentially limited to developing countries.

Dilated cardiomyopathy

Dilated cardiomyopathy describes the presence of left ventricular dilatation with or without the involvement of the right ventricle. Myocardial cells are also hypertrophied, with increased extracellular fibrosis. The condition may have a familial basis. Other causes include infective (usually viral) myocarditis, toxins and drugs such as alcohol and certain chemotherapies (eg doxorubicin) and systemic connective tissue diseases such as systemic lupus erythematosus and polyarteritis nodosa. Idiopathic dilated cardiomyopathy is diagnosed when all other causes have been excluded (Table 2.2).

The left ventricle is usually hypokinetic globally, resulting in impaired systolic function. Ventricular dilatation can produce atrial and ventricular arrhythmias and may also cause functional valvular regurgitation.

Table 2.2
Non-ischaemic causes of dilated cardiomyopathy

- *Familial*
- *Infectious*
  - viral (coxsackie B, cytomegalovirus, HIV)
  - rickettsia
  - bacteria (diphtheria)
  - mycobacteria
  - fungi
  - parasites (Chagas' disease, toxoplasmosis)
- *Toxins*
  - alcohol
  - cardiotoxic drugs (adriamycin, doxorubicin, zidovudine)
  - cocaine
  - metals (cobalt, mercury, lead)
- *Nutritional disease*
  - beriberi, kwashiorkor, pellagra
- *Endocrine disease*
  - myxoedema, thyrotoxicosis, acromegaly, phaeochromocytoma
- *Pregnancy*
- *Collagen disease*
  - connective tissue diseases (systemic lupus erythematosus, scleroderma, polyarteritis nodosa)
- *Neuromuscular disease*
  - Duchenne muscular dystrophy, myotonic dystrophy
- *Idiopathic*

Chronic alcohol abuse leads to dilated cardiomyopathy

Hypertrophic cardiomyopathy

Hypertrophic cardiomyopathy is normally regarded as an autosomal dominant inherited disease, although sporadic cases may occur. Classically, there is asymmetrical septal hypertrophy on echocardiography, which may be associated with aortic outflow obstruction (hypertrophic obstructive cardiomyopathy, HOCM) (Figure 2.3). Other rarer forms exist.

The outflow tract obstruction causes increased afterload. As with hypertension, the hypertrophic left ventricle is less compliant, with high end-diastolic pressures and reduced filling. There is a common association with

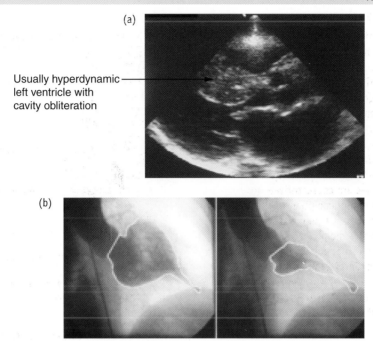

(a)

Usually hyperdynamic left ventricle with cavity obliteration

(b)

Figure 2.3
(a) Two-dimensional echocardiography and (b) left ventriculogram of a 35-year-old woman with hypertrophic cardiomyopathy. In (a), echocardiographic features include asymmetrical septal hypertrophy, systolic anterior motion of the anterior mitral valve leaflet and, on occasion, some mitral regurgitation.

atrial and ventricular arrhythmias, the latter leading to sudden cardiac death.

Restrictive and obliterative cardiomyopathies

Restrictive cardiomyopathy is characterized by a stiff and poorly compliant ventricle. This too is associated with abnormalities of diastolic function (relaxation) that limit ventricular filling.

The more common causes of restrictive cardiomyopathy in the west are infiltrative diseases including amyloidosis, sarcoidosis and haemochromatosis. Endomyocardial fibrosis is an important cause in developing countries. Endocardial fibrosis of the inflow tract of one or both ventricles, including the subvalvular regions, results in restriction of diastolic filling and cavity obliteration.

Valvular disease

The overall incidence of valvular disease has been steadily declining in the west, but it is still an important cause of heart failure in the developing countries, where rheumatic fever remains prevalent and untreated.

Heart failure is mainly due to mitral regurgitation or aortic stenosis (Figure 2.4). Mitral regurgitation leads to volume overload and resulting increased preload. On the other hand aortic stenosis leads to pressure overload, very much like hypertension and hypertrophic cardiomyopathy. Left ventricular hypertrophy eventually develops with aortic stenosis, and without valve replacement is associated with a poor prognosis. In contrast, patients with chronic mitral (or aortic) regurgitation generally decline in a slower and more progressive manner.

(a)

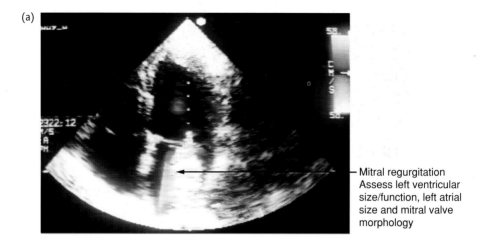

Mitral regurgitation
Assess left ventricular
size/function, left atrial
size and mitral valve
morphology

(b)

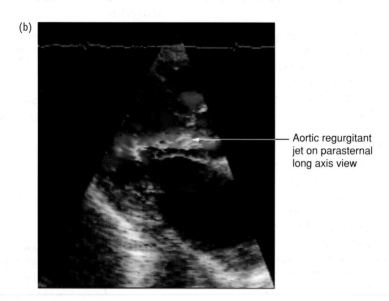

Aortic regurgitant
jet on parasternal
long axis view

Figure 2.4
Colour flow Doppler echocardiography of (a) severe mitral regurgitation and (b) severe aortic regurgitation.

Arrhythmias

Cardiac arrhythmias contribute to heart failure in various ways. Tachycardias dramatically reduce ventricular filling time in diastole. Myocardial oxygen demand is also increased, which may lead to ischaemia. If allowed to continue uncontrolled, tachycardia may lead to ventricular dilatation and systolic dysfunction, the so-called 'tachycardia-induced cardiomyopathy' (Figure 2.5). Bradycardias can result in a fall in cardiac output that is not

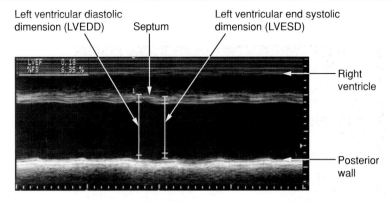

Left ventricular diastolic dimension (LVEDD)   Septum   Left ventricular end systolic dimension (LVESD)

Right ventricle

Posterior wall

Figure 2.5
M-mode echocardiography of a 50-year-old man admitted with fast atrial fibrillation showing left ventricular dilatation and severe dysfunction.

normally adequately compensated by increased stroke volume.

Both atrial and ventricular arrhythmias are more common among patients with heart failure and associated structural heart disease, including hypertensive patients with left ventricular hypertrophy. Ventricular arrhythmias may lead to a sudden deterioration in some patients and are a major cause of sudden death for patients with heart failure.

Atrial fibrillation is particularly important because of its common association with heart failure. Furthermore, atrial fibrillation is the commonest arrhythmia leading to hospitalization (Figure 2.6). The Hillingdon study found atrial fibrillation to be present in up to 30% of patients presenting for the first time with heart failure. Other studies have shown the prevalence of atrial fibrillation to be 6–50%, depending upon the severity of heart failure in the cohort of patients studied (Figure 2.7). The loss of atrial systole and active ventricular filling may be particularly crucial for patients with severe heart failure. Atrial fibrillation in patients with heart failure has been associated with increased mortality in some studies. Heart failure or left ventricular dysfunction increases the risk of stroke and

thromboembolism in patients with atrial fibrillation.

> Ventricular arrhythmias are a major cause of sudden death in patients with heart failure

- Miscellaneous 21%
- Conduction abnormalities 8%
- SSS 9%
- Premature beats 6%
- PSVT 6%
- Atrial flutter 4%
- Atrial fibrillation 34%
- VF 2%
- VT 10%

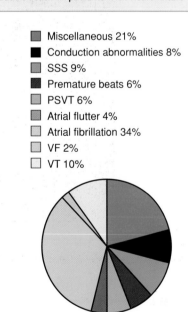

Figure 2.6
Hospitalizations for arrhythmia in the United States.
Adapted from Bialy D, Lehman MH, Schumacher DN *et al. J Am Coll Cardiol* 1992; **19**: 14A.

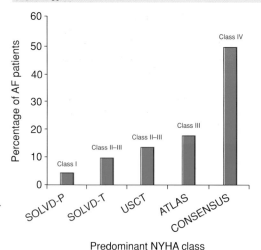

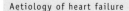

Figure 2.7
Atrial fibrillation in the major heart failure trials.

Alcohol and drugs

Alcohol contributes to at least 2–3% of chronic heart failure. Alcohol contributes to heart failure in several ways. It is directly cardiotoxic and can cause acute heart failure or heart failure as a result of arrhythmias, commonly atrial fibrillation. Chronic alcohol abuse leads to dilated cardiomyopathy (alcoholic heart muscle disease). Severe nutritional deficiency and thiamine deficiency accompanying alcoholism may sometimes be misdiagnosed as nutritional cardiac disease.

Certain drugs, particularly chemotherapeutic agents (for example, doxorubicin) and antiviral drugs (for example, zidovudine), are known to cause heart failure through direct toxic effects on the myocardium.

Other causes

Many conditions can give rise to heart failure despite normal myocardium and left ventricular function. Pericardial diseases and effusion (tamponade) can restrict sufficient filling in diastole (Figure 2.8).

'High output' heart failure, where cardiac output is inadequate despite normal contractility and filling pressures, is most often seen in patients with severe anaemia; thyrotoxicosis and septicaemia are other possible causes of failure. Infections may

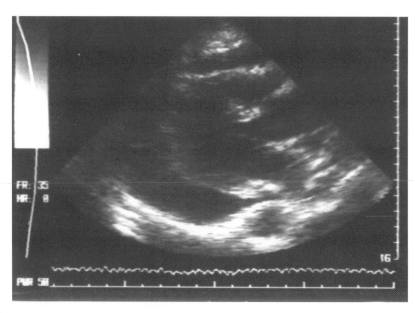

Figure 2.8
Two-dimensional echocardiogram showing large pericardial effusion.

cause acid–base disturbance, peripheral vasodilatation and tachycardia, resulting in acute heart failure (septicaemic shock).

Further reading

Levy D, Larson MG, Vasan RS *et al*. The progression from hypertension to congestive heart failure. *JAMA* 1996; **275**: 1557–62.

Lip GYH, Sarwar S, Ahmed I *et al*. A survey of heart failure in general practice. The west Birmingham heart failure project. *Eur J Gen Pract* 1997; **3**: 85–9.

Oakley C. Aetiology, diagnosis, investigation, and management of cardiomyopathies. *BMJ* 1997; **315**: 1520–4.

Teerlink JR, Goldhaber SZ, Pfeffer MA. An overview of contemporary etiologies of congestive heart failure. *Am Heart J* 1991; **121**: 1852–3.

3. Pathophysiology

Systolic dysfunction and diastolic dysfunction
Neurohormonal activation
Other noncardiovascular abnormalities in heart failure

Heart failure occurs when the heart fails to provide adequate circulation to metabolizing tissues in the body. It is characterized by abnormalities of cardiac and skeletal muscle and of renal function, as well as a complex pattern of neurohormonal activation.

Systolic dysfunction and diastolic dysfunction

Systolic dysfunction is present when there is impairment in left ventricular contractility, leading to a fall in cardiac output. This is the usual mechanism for most cases of nonvalvular heart failure. Impaired contractility may be confined to a segment of the left ventricle (such as following a myocardial infarct) or to the entire left ventricle (eg dilated cardiomyopathy and myocarditis). The fall in cardiac output activates several primitive compensatory mechanisms aimed at restoring the mechanical environment of the heart (Figure 3.1).

Diastolic dysfunction refers to impairment of diastolic ventricular filling which is usually a result of impaired myocardial relaxation secondary to increased stiffness in the ventricular wall and/or reduced left ventricular compliance. Infiltrative diseases such as amyloidosis are the best examples, although hypertension (with left ventricular hypertrophy), and hypertrophic cardiomyopathy are more common causes.

Most patients with heart failure exhibit both diastolic and systolic dysfunction. Isolated diastolic dysfunction (in the presence of normal ventricular systolic function) probably occurs in about 30–40% of patients with heart failure and is recognized increasingly in elderly patients and those with diabetes. It remains debatable whether or not isolated diastolic dysfunction is important prognostically or how it should ideally be managed.

Compensatory mechanisms in myocardial systolic dysfunction

When cardiac output falls, compensatory mechanisms are stimulated to provide circulatory support. Three compensatory mechanisms of importance are the Starling's mechanism, neurohormonal system stimulation and cardiac remodelling.

The heart initially increases stroke volume (cardiac output) by adapting to higher filling pressures and larger end-diastolic left ventricular volume. This is known as the Starling's mechanism. Progressive myocardial hypertrophy also develops, with or without ventricular dilatation, to sustain adequate systolic stress in the face of increasing end-diastolic pressures.

A host of neurohormonal changes also occur to promote peripheral vasoconstriction (angiotensin II) together with salt and water retention (aldosterone, vasopressin), and increase in heart rate and contractility (catecholamines) to maintain cardiac output. The ultimate result of persistent activation of these primitive neurohormones is the worsening of heart failure.

Both diastolic and systolic dysfunction are seen in most patients with heart failure

(a)

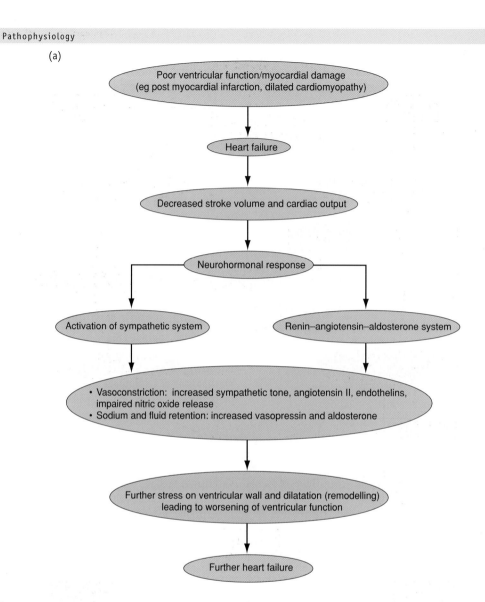

Figure 3.1
Pathophysiology of heart failure. (a) Neurohormonal mechanisms and compensatory mechanisms. (b) Drug therapy and pathophysiology of heart failure. (c) Determinants of ventricular function.

Neurohormonal activation

The neurohormonal systems that have been widely investigated include the renin–angiotensin–aldosterone system (RAAS), the sympathetic system, the natriuretic system and vasopressin. We are also starting to discover more about the endothelin system.

Renin–angiotensin–aldosterone system

Renal hypoperfusion stimulates the release of renin from the juxtaglomerular apparatus in the kidneys. Renin in turn stimulates the release of angiotensinogen, which is converted ultimately to the active and potent vasoconstrictor angiotensin II. Angiotensin II acts upon the

(b)

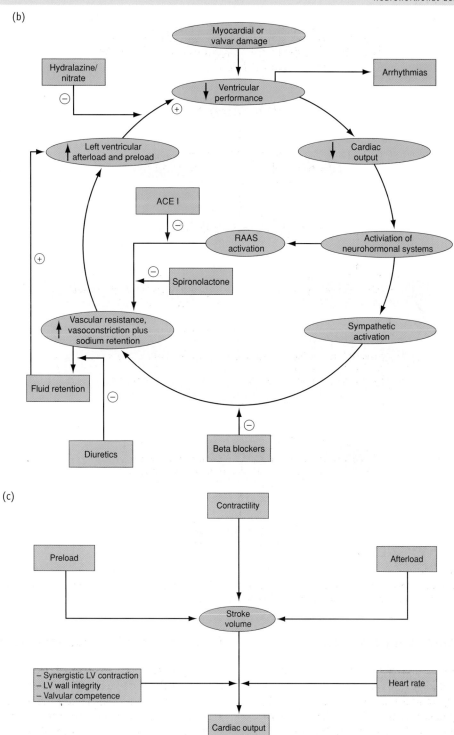

(c)

Figure 3.1 *continued*

efferent arterioles in the kidneys to increase glomerular filtration and upon the peripheral vessels to increase blood pressure.

Angiotensin II also stimulates noradrenaline release from sympathetic nerve terminals, inhibits vagal tone and promotes the release of aldosterone. Aldosterone acts upon the distal tubules of the kidneys to retain sodium and water while excreting potassium. This increases preload in the short term but contributes to fluid retention in the long term. Finally, angiotensin II promotes cardiac remodelling through its effects on cardiac myocytes (Figure 3.2).

Sympathetic nervous system

Plasma noradrenaline level increases early in the development of heart failure. The sympathetic nervous system is activated through baroreceptors in response to falls in blood pressure and cardiac output. In the short term, increased catecholamines stimulate heart rate and myocardial contractility via beta-1 receptors and vasoconstriction peripherally via alpha receptors. Noradrenaline also activates the renin–angiotensin–aldosterone system.

Persistent noradrenaline and inotropic stimulation of the failing heart causes cardiac

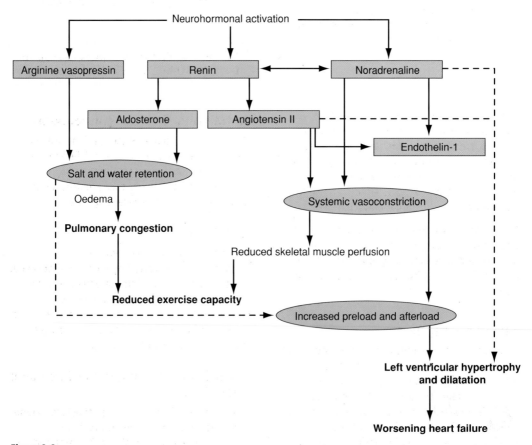

Figure 3.2
Deleterious effects of chronic neurohormonal activation.

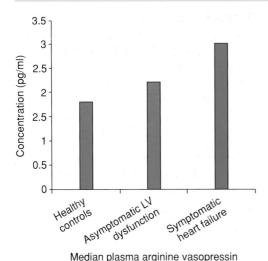

Figure 3.3

Elevated plasma circulating levels of arginine vasopressin (AVP) in patients with asymptomatic and symptomatic left ventricular dysfunction.

ventricles in humans. Both ANP and BNP induce sodium excretion and vasodilatation. Hence, they act essentially to counterbalance the actions of the RAAS and the sympathetic nervous system.

Recent interest has focused upon developing natriuretic peptide agonists and inhibitors of their breakdown enzyme, neural endopeptidase. The natriuretic peptides may prove to be most useful as diagnostic and prognostic markers in chronic heart failure. Plasma concentrations of *N*-terminal pro-atrial natriuretic peptide and BNP seem to be good indicators of asymptomatic left ventricular dysfunction, while raised plasma concentrations of *N*-terminal and *C*-terminal atrial natriuretic peptide and of brain natriuretic peptide are independent predictors of mortality in patients with chronic heart failure.

> Natriuretic peptides may be useful diagnostic and prognostic markers in chronic heart failure

myocyte apoptosis, hypertrophy and focal myocardial necrosis. It also predisposes the heart to arrhythmias, which may lead to sudden cardiac deaths. Furthermore, down-regulation of beta receptors in the heart results in attenuation of sympathetic effects on the heart and further catecholamine elevation.

Noradrenaline concentration in asymptomatic left ventricular dysfunction is a strong and independent predictor of symptomatic chronic heart failure and subsequent mortality (Figure 3.3).

Natriuretic peptides

Three natriuretic peptides are known. All are of similar structure and exert a wide range of effects on the heart, kidneys and central nervous system. The atrial natriuretic peptide (ANP) is released from the atria in response to stretch. The B-type natriuretic peptide, previously known as brain natriuretic peptide (BNP), is released predominantly from the

Antidiuretic hormone (vasopressin)

Antidiuretic hormone concentrations are also increased in severe chronic heart failure and may be due to iatrogenic diuretic use. Antidiuretic hormone further predisposes to free water retention and worsening oedema.

Endothelins

The endothelins are very powerful vasocontrictors secreted by vascular endothelial cells, and are responsible for arteriolar tone modulation. Abnormal plasma levels of endothelin-1 have been found to correlate with severity of heart failure and are also markers for frequent hospitalization and death.

Other hormonal mechanisms in chronic heart failure

The kallikrein–kinin system is stimulated along with the RAAS in the kidneys to form bradykinin, which promotes natriuresis and vasodilatation. Bradykinin also stimulates increased production of prostaglandins (PGE2 and PGI2), which protect the glomerular microcirculation by dilating the afferent arterioles. This system counteracts the RAAS.

Finally, raised levels of inflammatory cytokines such as tumour necrosis factor (TNF) have been found in chronic heart failure. Their precise role(s) are uncertain but they have been implicated in endothelial dysfunction in chronic heart failure.

Other noncardiovascular abnormalities in heart failure

Vasculature

The vascular endothelium is not an inert layer of cells but plays an important role in the regulation of vascular tone, releasing relaxing and contracting factors under basal conditions or during exercise. Impairment of endothelial function leads to increased concentrations of endothelin (a powerful vasoconstrictor) and a reduction in the level of nitric oxide (endothelium derived relaxing factor), resulting in vasoconstriction and increased afterload.

Numerous factors have been known to cause endothelial damage and dysfunction, including noradrenaline, angiotensin II and TNF-alpha. There is emerging evidence that impaired endothelial function in chronic heart failure may be improved with exercise training and drug treatment, such as the use of ACE inhibitors.

> Endothelial function in chronic heart failure may be improved with exercise training

Skeletal muscle changes

One of the hallmarks of chronic heart failure is muscle weakness leading to lethargy and easy fatigability. This is due to vasoconstriction leading to reduced blood flow to skeletal muscle with consequent reduction in muscle metabolism, mass and function.

Myocardial remodelling

The myocardium adapts to increased preload and afterload in the long term by myocyte hypertrophy. This leads to hypertrophy of the

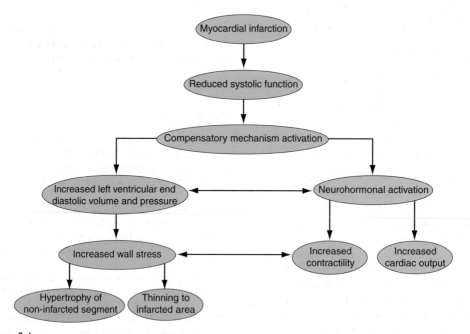

Figure 3.4
Process of ventricular remodelling following myocardial infarction.

left ventricle and allows for sufficient systolic stress to overcome the increased preload. In hypertension and outflow tract obstruction such as aortic stenosis, concentric hypertrophy usually develops. After extensive myocardial infarction, there is usually regional eccentric hypertrophy of the non-infarcted area, with thinning and dilatation of the infarct zone. Dilatation can also occur with sustained preload and afterload (Figure 3.4). These structural myocyte alterations are known as cardiac remodelling and are influenced by increased noradrenaline and angiotensin II.

Myocardial hibernation and stunning

There are two conditions whereby impaired myocardial contractility may be reversible. In post-ischaemic dysfunction, there may be a delay in recovery of myocardial function despite restoration of coronary blood flow and in the absence of irreversible damage. This is known as 'myocardial stunning'. During a period of stunning, left ventricular ejection fraction may be significantly impaired until recovery occurs. By definition, this transient contractile dysfunction is fully reversible provided sufficient time is allowed, although the duration of the dysfunction may greatly exceed that of the antecedent ischaemia.

In contrast, 'hibernating myocardium' refers to persistent myocardial dysfunction at rest, secondary to reduced myocardial perfusion, although the myocytes remain viable; this condition may, however, be improved following the restoration of coronary blood flow.

Both conditions may be identified by resting and stress echocardiography, thallium scintigraphy and positron emission tomography. Revascularization may improve overall myocardial function.

Prothrombotic or hypercoagulable state

It is well recognized that patients with congestive heart failure are at an increased risk of stroke and venous thromboembolism. Nevertheless, in large heart failure trials stroke, thromboembolism and myocardial infarction have generally been regarded to be endpoints of secondary importance as compared with mortality or hospital readmissions. It may well have been that the incidence of thrombotic events has been underestimated. The problem of thrombus formation (thrombogenesis) in heart failure may therefore be much more significant than is currently recognized.

The pathophysiology of thrombogenesis in heart failure could well be explained in the context of Virchow's original triad. In addition to 'abnormal flow' through low cardiac output, dilated cardiac chambers and poor contractility, patients with heart failure also demonstrate abnormalities of haemostasis and platelets (that is 'abnormal blood constituents') and endothelial dysfunction ('vessel wall abnormalities'). These abnormalities contribute to a prothrombotic or hypercoagulable state, which increases the risk of thrombosis in patients with heart failure and impaired left ventricular systolic function.

> The significance of thrombogenesis in heart failure currently may be underestimated

Further reading

Grossman W. Diastolic dysfunction in congestive heart failure. *N Engl J Med* 1991; **325**: 1557–64.

Lip GYH, Gibbs CR. Does heart failure confer a hypercoagulable state? Virchow's triad revisited. *J Am Coll Cardiol* 1999; **33**: 1424–6.

Love MP, McMurray JJV. Endothelin in heart failure: a promising therapeutic target. *Heart* 1997; **77**: 93–4.

McDonagh TA, Robb SD, Murdoch DR *et al*. Biochemical detection of left ventricular systolic dysfunction. *Lancet* 1998; **351**: 9–13.

Packer M. The neurohormonal hypothesis: a theory to explain the mechanisms of disease progression in heart failure. *J Am Coll Cardiol* 1992; **20**: 248–54.

Wilkins MR, Redondo J, Brown LA. The natriuretic-peptide family. *Lancet* 1997; **349**: 1307–10.

4. Clinical features

Symptoms
Physical signs
Clinical diagnosis and clinical scoring systems
Classification of severity
Complications of heart failure

Heart failure is a syndrome that normally comprises fatigue, dyspnoea and fluid retention (oedema) (Figure 4.1). These and other symptoms of heart failure (Table 4.1) are rather nonspecific, however. Making a diagnosis by presenting clinical features alone is therefore not very accurate.

Table 4.1
Symptoms and signs in heart failure

- *Symptoms*
  - Dyspnoea
  - Orthopnoea
  - Paroxysmal nocturnal dyspnoea
  - Reduced exercise tolerance, lethargy and fatigue
  - Nocturnal cough
  - Wheeze
  - Ankle swelling
  - Anorexia
- *Signs*
  - Cachexia and muscle wasting
  - Tachycardia
  - Pulsus alternans
  - Elevated jugular venous pressure
  - Displaced apex beat
  - Right ventricular heave
  - Crepitations or wheeze
  - Third heart sound
  - Oedema
  - Hepatomegaly (tender)
  - Ascites

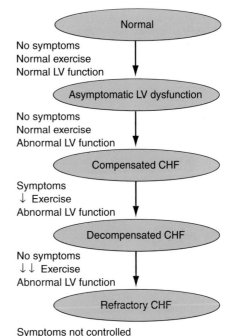

Figure 4.1
Evolution of the clinical stages of heart failure.
CHF= congestive heart failure; LV= left ventricular.

Symptoms

Dyspnoea

Dyspnoea or breathlessness is a common symptom of heart failure. Patients may complain of breathlessness on lying flat (orthopnoea), on minimal activity or on moderate exertion. The symptoms associated with heart failure are incorporated into the New York Heart Association (NYHA) classification of the functional severity of the condition (Table 4.2).

Exertional dyspnoea is a relatively nonspecific symptom of heart failure, however, as it is quite common in the general population. Orthopnoea is more specific but is not always present in heart failure, and therefore has little predictive value. Paroxysmal nocturnal dyspnoea refers to 'waking up with intense breathlessness and needing to sit up or stand'. It is caused by

Table 4.2
Classification of functional severity of heart failure
according to the New York Heart Association (NYHA)

- *Class I: asymptomatic*
  No limitation in physical activity despite
  presence of heart disease

- *Class II: mild*
  Slight limitation in physical activity. Symptoms
  only with moderate activity – for example,
  walking on steep inclines and several flights of
  steps. Patients in this group can continue to
  have an almost normal lifestyle and
  employment

- *Class III: moderate*
  Symptoms occur with mild activity or activities
  associated with daily living – for example,
  walking on the level, putting on clothes

- *Class IV: severe*
  Unable to carry out any physical activity
  without symptoms. Patients are breathless at
  rest and mostly housebound

Nocturnal angina (or chest pains typical of
cardiac ischaemia) may also result from
increased left ventricular filling pressures and
may indicate poorly controlled heart failure.

Fatigue and lethargy

Structural and metabolic changes that occur
in skeletal muscle in heart failure lead to easy
fatigability. Cerebral perfusion is also reduced,
and when accompanied by frequently
disturbed nights can cause daytime
somnolence and confusion. Depression may
also be a factor in chronic heart failure,
particularly for patients who are dependent or
not ambulatory.

> Depression may be a significant factor in
> dependent patients

Oedema

Lower limb oedema is another common
presenting feature. It is due to fluid retention
and predominantly to right sided failure. There
may be sacral oedema, particularly in less
ambulatory patients confined to bed. Ascites
(abdominal swelling with shifting dullness) and

increased left ventricular filling pressures
secondary to nocturnal fluid redistribution and
enhanced renal reabsorption. It is more common
than orthopnoea in heart failure and more
specific than exertional dyspnoea; it therefore
has a high predictive value (Table 4.3).

Table 4.3
Positive predictive value of presenting symptoms and signs for presence of heart failure (ejection
fraction <40%) in 1306 patients with coronary artery disease

Clinical features	Sensitivity (%)	Specificity (%)	Positive predictive value (%)
History			
● shortness of breath	66	52	23
● orthopnoea	21	81	2
● paroxysmal nocturnal dyspnoea	33	76	26
● history of oedema	23	80	22
Examination			
● tachycardia (>100 beats/min)	7	99	6
● crepitations	13	91	27
● oedema (on examination)	10	93	3
● gallop (S3)	31	95	61
● neck vein distension	10	97	2
● cardiomegaly on chest X-ray	62	67	32

From Harlan WR, Oberman A, Grimm R, Rosati RA. *Ann Intern Med* 1977; **86**: 133–8.

liver congestion (enlarged liver with tenderness) are also features of right sided failure. Both lower limb oedema and ascites are common in other conditions and therefore have low specificity and predictive values.

Weight changes

Fluid retention increases the total body weight of the patient, and daily measurement of weight is therefore often taken to indicate the degree of success in achieving fluid loss. This can be confounded in the patient with severe chronic heart failure, however, whose body weight may be affected both by increased fluid retention and by losses through cardiac cachexia.

Cardiac cachexia results in part from muscle atrophy and breakdown (related to lack of use, reduced skeletal muscle perfusion and metabolic changes) but also from anorexia and malabsorption (due to bowel oedema and liver congestion).

Physical signs

Many patients with heart failure present with few clinical signs, even though clinical symptoms may be evident. Some signs are also difficult to interpret. However, they are generally more specific than heart failure symptoms.

Clinical signs such as elevated jugular venous pressure, pulmonary crepitations, a displaced apex beat or a third heart sound are very specific for heart failure but lack sensitivity. For example, pulmonary crepitations can be found in patients with pulmonary fibrosis, pneumonia and emphysema. Tachycardia, gallop rhythm and lower limb oedema are also relatively insensitive. Lower limb oedema is commonly found in elderly people and those who are less mobile.

Certain signs related to the cause of heart failure may be present. For example, the patient may look very pale (anaemia), or may have a pyrexia (or hypothermia) from sepsis, or an arrhythmia. Patients with thyrotoxicosis may be very thin and sweaty, with a fine tremor of the hands. Chronic alcohol abuse leading to heart failure may also cause liver cirrhosis with all the stigmata of

chronic liver failure. These signs can help in diagnosing heart failure. Other precipitating causes of heart failure, such as heart murmur or raised blood pressure, should also be sought.

Clinical diagnosis and clinical scoring systems

In general, if a patient presents with appropriate symptoms plus some of the physical signs mentioned above, a diagnosis of heart failure may be made. This should be confirmed by objective measurements such as echocardiography, nuclear imaging or contrast ventriculography.

> Heart failure is difficult to diagnose, and ventricular dysfunction may not be clinically evident

Several epidemiological studies, including the Framingham heart study, have used clinical scoring systems to define heart failure, although the use of these systems is not recommended for routine clinical practice.

The ESC guidelines for the diagnosis of heart failure recommend as indicators the presence of typical symptoms (dyspnoea, lethargy, ankle swelling, etc) and objective confirmation of cardiac dysfunction at rest. Where the diagnosis remains in doubt, a response to treatment directed towards alleviation of heart failure makes the diagnosis more likely.

European Society of Cardiology criteria for diagnosis of heart failure

To satisfy the diagnosis of heart failure, there must be:

- Appropriate symptoms of heart failure
- Objective evidence of cardiac dysfunction
- Appropriate response to relevant treatment, in cases of doubt
- Echocardiography – the most practical tool to demonstrate cardiac dysfunction

Adapted from *Eur Heart J* 1995; **16**: 741–51.

Table 4.4
Killip class scoring and corresponding hospital mortality

Class	Clinical features	Hospital mortality (%)
Class I	No signs of left ventricular dysfunction	6
Class II	S3 gallop with or without mild to moderate pulmonary congestion	30
Class III	Acute severe pulmonary oedema	40
Class IV	Shock syndrome	80–90

Adapted from Killip T, Kimball JT. *Am J Cardiol* 1967; **20**: 457–64.

Heart failure may be diagnosed if a patient exhibits appropriate symptoms plus some physical signs.

Classification of severity

Many systems of classification of severity of heart failure have been formulated, of which that produced by the New York Heart Association (NYHA) is most widely used. This measures heart failure according to functional (symptomatic) status and exercise capacity (Table 4.2).

Heart failure can also be classified using echocardiographic criteria or according to presence of clinical features of heart failure (Killip class scoring) (Table 4.4).

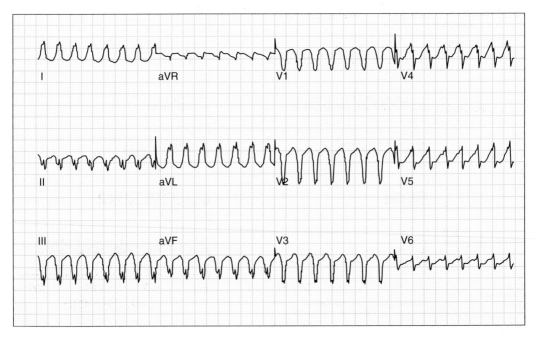

Figure 4.2
ECG tracing of a 52-year-old man with sustained ventricular tachycardia one hour after presenting with acute myocardial infarction.

Complications of heart failure

Arrhythmias

Ventricular arrhythmias

Patients with ventricular dysfunction commonly exhibit ventricular extrasystoles on electrocardiography. Patients with end-stage heart failure are at increased risk of developing malignant ventricular arrhythmias. For patients with ischaemic heart disease these arrhythmias often have re-entrant mechanisms in scarred myocardial tissue. An episode of sustained ventricular tachycardia (Figure 4.2) is a predictor of recurrent ventricular arrhythmias and sudden cardiac death.

Factors that predispose to ventricular arrhythmias in heart failure include myocardial ischaemia (recurrent angina, myocardial infarction),

electrolyte abnormalities (hyper- or hypokalaemia, hypomagnesaemia) and drugs (including antiarrhythmics, digoxin and psychotropic drugs). These predisposing factors also cause polymorphic ventricular tachycardia (*torsades de pointes*).

Atrial fibrillation

Atrial fibrillation (AF) is common in heart failure. In the Echocardiographic Heart of England Screening study, definite heart failure was associated with atrial fibrillation in 33% of cases. The loss of atrial systole and presence of rapid ventricular rate in AF may precipitate or exacerbate heart failure. Predisposing factors of AF should therefore be looked for to rule out important causes such as thyrotoxicosis, mitral valve disease and sinus node disease. Patients with atrial fibrillation and heart failure have a greatly increased risk of stroke and increased mortality.

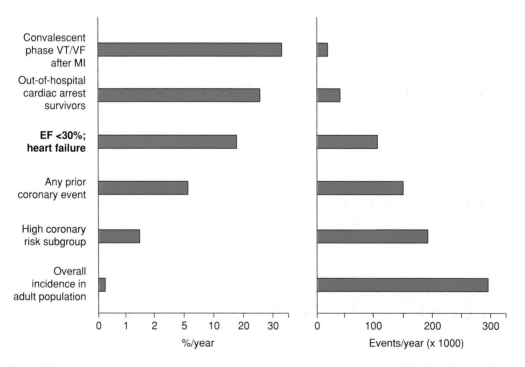

Figure 4.3
Percentage per year of sudden cardiac death in patients with heart failure (ejection fraction <30%) compared to overall adult population in the United States and other high-risk subgroups. Adapted from Myeburg RJ, Kessler KM, Castellanos A. *Circulation* 1992; **85** (I Suppl): I2–10.

Sudden death

The incidence of sudden cardiac death in (severe) heart failure patients with ejection fractions <30% is approximately 15–20% per year (Figure 4.3).

Sudden cardiac deaths are usually presumed to be due to ventricular arrhythmias. Some autopsy studies have revealed the presence of fresh coronary thrombus, suggesting that acute coronary occlusion may have been the primary event. The cause of death is often uncertain, especially as the patient usually dies before reaching hospital.

Stroke and thromboembolism

Congestive heart failure in sinus rhythm itself also predisposes to stroke and thromboembolism, with an overall estimated annual incidence of approximately 2%. The emboli presumably originate from left ventricular thrombi (Figure 4.4).

Factors that predispose to ventricular thrombus formation include regional wall motion abnormalities, presence of ventricular aneurysm, low cardiac output and atrial fibrillation. These conditions give rise to relative stasis of blood in dilated cardiac chambers.

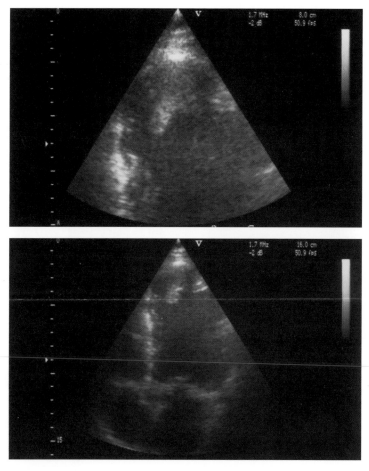

Figure 4.4
Two-dimensional echocardiography in the apical four-chamber view (top image magnified) of a 42-year-old patient with recent anterior segment myocardial infarction, showing a protruding thrombus in the left ventricle with a pedunculated stalk.

> Patients with atrial fibrillation and heart failure have an increased risk of stroke

The risk of stroke is associated with severity of heart failure, with patients at NYHA class IV carrying a 4% increased risk of stroke. Furthermore, there appears to be an 18% increased risk for every 5% reduction in ejection fraction (as measured by echocardiography). The presence of atrial fibrillation also increases the risk of stroke considerably. Finally, patients with heart failure tend to be less mobile and this may put them at increased risk of venous thromboembolism.

Noncardiovascular complications

Uraemia reflects poor renal perfusion and may result from low cardiac output and renal vasoconstriction. Electrolyte disturbances are very common and may be due to the actions of neurohormones in heart failure as well as diuretic therapy.

The patient with advanced heart failure may also be jaundiced and show impaired liver function tests including elevated clotting times. Liver failure is usually due to increased venous pressures resulting in liver congestion and cirrhosis. Abdominal discomfort, right upper quadrant abdominal tenderness, anorexia, nausea and vomiting are therefore quite common. Malabsorption secondary to reduced internal blood flow results in hypoalbuminaemia and further oedema.

Further reading

Dargie HJ, McMurray JVV. Diagnosis and management of heart failure. *BMJ* 1994; **308**: 321–8.

Task Force on Heart Failure of the European Society of Cardiology. Guidelines for the diagnosis of heart failure. *Eur Heart J* 1995; **16**: 741–51.

5. Investigation of heart failure

Chest X-ray
Twelve-lead electrocardiography
Echocardiography
Haematology and biochemistry
Radionuclide methods
Cardiac catheterization and
myocardial biopsy

Investigations into the diagnosis and cause of heart failure are usually necessary, but this step should take place only after careful clinical assessment.

Basic essential cardiological investigative tools for investigating heart failure include chest radiography, 12-lead electrocardiography (ECG), full blood count and serum biochemistry, including renal function, glucose, liver function and thyroid function tests. Echocardiography is the single most important non-invasive method and should ideally be performed in any patient suspected of having heart failure. Further investigations may include radionuclide imaging, cardiopulmonary exercise testing, cardiac catheterization and, rarely, myocardial biopsy.

Chest X-ray

The chest X-ray examination is most useful in detecting pulmonary congestion in acute or decompensated left-sided heart failure and in excluding respiratory causes of dypsnoea. Pulmonary venous congestion is initially evident as prominent and dilated vasculature in the upper zones (referred to as upper lobe diversion or congestion). As pulmonary venous

pressure increases further, usually above 20 mmHg, fluid may be present in the fissures (Kerley B lines and clear horizontal fissure). At higher pressures, frank pulmonary or alveolar oedema develops with or without pleural effusion.

The chest X-ray is therefore also useful to guide responses to treatment and control of heart failure. It should be noted that pulmonary oedema can occur in other conditions such as renal failure and acute respiratory distress syndrome.

In chronic heart failure, cardiac enlargement (cardiothoracic ratio >50%) may be present. This may be due to left or right ventricle dilatation, left ventricular hypertrophy, and occasionally a pericardial effusion.

Twelve-lead electrocardiograph

The 12-lead ECG tracing in patients with heart failure commonly shows nonspecific ST and T segment abnormalities, left ventricular hypertrophy or bundle branch block. Pathological Q waves suggestive of previous myocardial infarctions and atrial fibrillation are also common.

The ECG is fairly specific in identifying heart failure (~60%) and reliable at excluding cardiac dysfunction if normal, with about 94% sensitivity and 98% negative predictive value. A normal ECG therefore makes it unlikely that the patient has heart failure secondary to left ventricular systolic dysfunction. The combination of a normal chest X-ray and a normal ECG makes a cardiac cause of dyspnoea improbable.

Echocardiography

Echocardiography provides an objective assessment of cardiac structure and function. It allows for identification of valvular diseases, pericardial diseases (pericardial effusions) and myocardial regional wall motion abnormality (ischaemic heart disease).

Ideally, almost all patients with symptoms or signs of heart failure, or with dyspnoea associated with a heart murmur or atrial fibrillation, should have an echocardiogram. Patients at risk of developing left ventricular dysfunction (eg following extensive myocardial infarct particularly involving the anterior wall), with poorly controlled hypertension, and arrhythmias should also be referred for echocardiographic examination.

The left ventricular function can be estimated from calculation of the left ventricular ejection fraction (LVEF) and/or fractional shortening (Figure 5.1). The LVEF has been shown to correlate well with outcome and survival for patients with heart failure. Certain conditions may make estimation of left ventricular function by LVEF less accurate: these include the presence of atrial fibrillation and regional wall motion abnormalities.

In such patients, it would be more useful to assess overall wall motion index. The left ventricle can be divided into 16 segments, which correspond roughly to anatomical

coronary artery perfusion and which are agreed universally. Abnormalities in wall motion are viewed and recorded for each segment as hypokinetic (reduced systolic contraction), akinetic (no systolic contraction) or dyskinetic (abnormalities of direction or timing of contraction, or both). In practice, left ventricular function is usually estimated from eyeballing the left ventricle in all standard views and is therefore subjective.

Echocardiography is also useful for determining the presence of diastolic dysfunction and assessment of the right ventricular function. The thromboembolic risk of cardiogenic origin can also be estimated (for example, if mural thrombus is present). Finally, valvular lesions can be detected and assessed for their severity.

A common valvular abnormality among patients with heart failure and left ventricular dilatation is mitral regurgitation. In functional mitral incompetence, the valve is morphologically normal and the incompetence

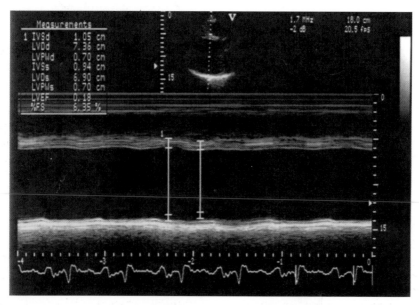

Figure 5.1
M-mode echocardiography of a 56-year-old patient following repair of mitral regurgitation showing a poorly contracting and dilated left ventricle.

is the result of annular dilatation. This can be distinguished from primary heart valve disease. Modern techniques in echocardiography such as Doppler and colour flow studies have vastly improved the sensitivity of identifying valvular diseases. Transoesophageal echocardiography is very useful for the detailed assessment of the atria, valves, pulmonary veins and any cardiac masses, including thrombi, and where the transthoracic window is limited.

> Echocardiography provides an objective assessment of cardiac structure and function

In recent years, increasing numbers of cardiology departments are beginning to offer open access echocardiography facilities so that general practitioners can refer patients with suspected heart failure. Although large scale screening is still costly, there is evidence that these services have resulted in earlier initiation of ACE inhibitors in heart failure, and with fewer subsequent hospital admissions.

Haematology and biochemistry

Routine haematology and biochemistry tests are needed to exclude anaemia, thyroid dysfunction and other important pre-existing metabolic abnormalities as contributory causes of heart failure. Where acute myocardial infarction is suspected, cardiac enzymes should also be analysed. Liver function tests can give an indication of hepatic involvement secondary to liver congestion.

Renal function and electrolytes may be abnormal in heart failure for various reasons. Renal function (serum creatinine) may be impaired as a result of renal hypoperfusion, use of high dose diuretics or ACE inhibitors in bilateral renal artery stenosis.

Diuretics, reduction in sodium intake and persistently elevated levels of neurohormones may lead to excess sodium loss. Water retention may also bring about a state of dilutional hyponatraemia. Many of these changes occur at end-stage heart failure, and hyponatraemia is therefore a marker of the severity of chronic heart failure.

Hypokalaemia occurs when high dose diuretics are used without potassium supplementation or potassium sparing agents. Hyperkalaemia can also occur in severe congestive heart failure with a low glomerular filtration rate, particularly with the concurrent use of ACE inhibitors and potassium sparing diuretics. Both hypokalaemia and hyperkalaemia increase the risk of cardiac arrhythmias, together with hypomagnesaemia, which is also associated with long term diuretic treatment.

Biochemical markers for diagnosis and prognosis of heart failure are currently being developed. At the time of writing, atrial and B-type natriuretic peptides are the most promising of these, although more work is needed before they can be used routinely in clinical practice.

Radionuclide methods

Radionuclide imaging allows for images to be obtained for assessment of global left and right ventricular function in patients where the scope of echocardiography is limited. In multigated ventriculography (MUGA), 16 or 32 frames are acquired for every heart beat and are synchronized using the ECG (Figure 5.2). It is possible to measure ejection fraction, systolic filling rate, diastolic emptying rate and wall motion abnormalities during rest and following stress with this method.

Stress studies may be performed using graded physical exercise or pharmacologically induced stress, usually with adenosine, dipyridamole or dobutamine. This method is particularly useful for identifying areas of myocardial infarction, reversible ischaemia suitable for revascularization, and the presence of myocardial stunning and hibernation.

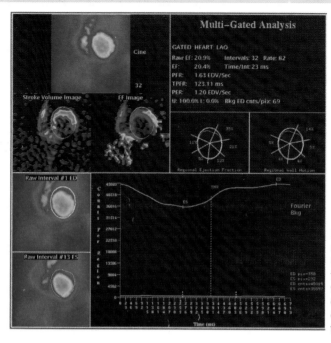

Figure 5.2
Multigated analysis (MUGA) using tetrofosmin of a patient with ischaemic cardiomyopathy. The calculated ejection fraction here was 20.4%.

Cardiac catheterization and myocardial biopsy

Angiography should be considered for patients with recurrent ischaemic chest pain associated with heart failure and in those with evidence of severe reversible ischaemia or hibernating myocardium. Cardiac catheterization of the left heart can show global or segmental impairment of function or a ventricular aneurysm (Figure 5.3), as well as assessing end-diastolic pressures.

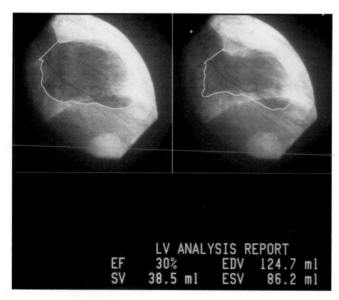

Figure 5.3
Ventriculography of a 73-year-old patient revealing a dyskinetic apical segment (apical aneurysm) when comparing views at end-diastole (left) and end-systole (right).

Right heart catheterization, on the other hand, allows for assessment of the right sided pressures (right atrium, right ventricle and pulmonary arteries) and pulmonary artery capillary wedge pressure, in addition to oxygen saturation.

Myocardial biopsy is used only in more difficult cases where there is diagnostic doubt; for example, in restrictive and infiltrating cardiomyopathies (amyloid heart disease, sarcoidosis), myocarditis and pericardial disease.

Echocardiography is the single most important non-invasive method of cardiological investigation

Further reading

ACC/AHA Task Force Report. Guidelines for the evaluation and management of heart failure. *J Am Coll Cardiol* 1995; **26**:1376–98.

6. Non-drug management

Counselling and education
Contraceptive advice
Lifestyle measures
Immunization and antibiotic prophylaxis
Diet and nutrition
Exercise and rehabilitation
Surgery and special procedures

Nonpharmacological measures are an essential part of the management plan for patients with heart failure (Table 6.1). Simple measures such as stopping smoking, losing weight and avoiding winter infections (for example, by the use of influenza and pneumococcal vaccinations) can prevent acute on chronic exacerbations of heart failure. A multidisciplinary approach to heart failure management, including input from the cardiologist, general practitioner, specialist nurse, dietician and (occasionally) clinical psychologist, may help in providing a comprehensive 'heart failure service'.

Counselling and education

Patients with chronic heart failure should be given the opportunity to ask about and understand their condition. Simple explanations about the symptoms and signs of heart failure, including details of drug and other treatment strategies, go a long way in improving patient compliance and morale in a chronic illness with poor prognosis. Patients can be instructed to monitor their weight and look out for signs of worsening heart failure (such as increasing ankle oedema).

Contraceptive advice

Women with severe heart failure should be counselled to avoid pregnancy, as in these patients the risk of maternal mortality is high with pregnancy and childbirth. Newer oral contraceptive pills are generally safer and carry a lower risk of thromboembolism, although caution is needed in patients with previous venous thromboembolism. Intra-uterine devices are also safe in women without valvular disease (risk of infection).

Lifestyle measures

Patients should be encouraged to continue their regular work where appropriate and to participate in social events.

Smoking

Patients who smoke must stop. Cigarette smoking increases the risk of coronary artery disease, reduces cardiac output and reduces lung function and capacity in patients already troubled by dyspnoea. Furthermore, smoking can have a vasoconstrictive effect, thus being detrimental to efforts to introduce vasodilator therapy in such patients.

Alcohol

Abstinence from alcohol is most important for patients with alcohol-induced dilated cardiomyopathy. Alcohol is directly toxic to the myocardium and may induce arrhythmias (especially atrial fibrillation) and hypertension.

In patients with alcohol-induced heart disease, abstinence usually results in improvement. In general, alcohol consumption should be restricted to moderate levels, given the myocardial depressant properties of alcohol.

> Simply stopping smoking, losing weight and avoiding winter infections can prevent exacerbations of heart failure

Immunization and antibiotic prophylaxis

Influenza and pneumococcal vaccinations are now recommended for patients with chronic heart failure. Antibiotic prophylaxis for dental and other surgical procedures is mandatory for patients with valvular disease and prosthetic heart valves.

Diet and nutrition

Adequate and appropriate nutritional balance is important for chronic illnesses. Patients with cardiac cachexia should be recommended a higher-energy diet supplemented with essential vitamins. On the other hand, more obese patients should be encouraged to lose weight to within 10% of their optimal body weight.

Patients should furthermore be advised to cut down on daily salt intake by avoiding salt-rich foods such as cheese, crisps, sausages and tinned or smoked products.

Patients with severe heart failure and features of volume overload who are not responding well to diuretics may have been negating the effects of diuretics by drinking excess water. Such patients should have their daily fluid intake monitored, and if it is excessive, be instructed to restrict their fluid allowance to 1.5–2 litres a day.

Exercise training and rehabilitation

Exercise training has been shown to improve patient symptoms and functional capacity. Hence, all patients with chronic stable heart failure should be encouraged to participate in a supervised, simple exercise programme. Indeed, chronic immobility may contribute to loss of muscle mass in heart failure as well as causing generalized physical deconditioning.

Regular exercise has the potential to halt this process while exerting beneficial autonomic effects (with reduced sympathetic activity and enhanced vagal tone). Large prospective clinical trials will establish whether exercise training in chronic stable heart failure improves prognosis and reduces mortality.

> Exercise training can improve both symptoms and functional capacity

A word of caution: patients should be aware of their limits and increase their exercise gradually. Excessive strain and fatigue should be avoided. Patients with ischaemic heart disease should also stop if their angina is provoked at short distances, while extreme unsupervised exercise may be harmful for patients with symptomatic hypertrophic cardiomyopathy or aortic stenosis.

Table 6.1
Nonpharmacological measures for the management of heart failure

Counselling: Education and advice about disease, objectives of treatment and self-help strategies

Diet: Maintaining a low-fat, low-salt and balanced diet. Diabetic patients should also observe a sugar-free diet and obese patients should be encouraged to lose weight. Patients with cardiac cachexia may require high-energy or protein diets

Fluid: Oral fluid intake may need to be restricted to 1–1.5 litres/day in patients with fluid overload who are resistant to diuretics

Smoking and alcohol: Patients must stop smoking. General advice on alcohol consumption may be given, but patients with alcohol-induced cardiomyopathy must observe strict abstention

Exercise: Regular and graduated exercise should be encouraged

Vaccination: Patients should consider influenza and pneumococcal vaccinations

Surgery and special procedures

Any reversible or treatable causes of heart failure should be managed appropriately to reduce or halt progression of heart failure. Secondary prevention of ischaemic heart disease is important. Percutaneous coronary angioplasty (PTCA) and coronary artery bypass grafting (CABG) should be offered to patients who would benefit from revascularization.

Valve replacement or repair should be considered for any patients with haemodynamically important primary valvular disease. Patients with resistant ventricular arrhythmias or bradycardias with haemodynamic instability should receive an implantable defibrillator or permanent pacemaker respectively.

Patients with acute or decompensated heart failure requiring support may benefit from the short term use of ventricular assist devices or intra-aortic balloon pumping.

Finally, younger patients (<60 years of age) with severe end-stage heart failure should be considered for cardiac transplantation. At the time of writing, cardiac transplantation offers a one-year survival of about 90% and a 10-year survival of 50–60%.

7. Drug therapy

Diuretics
ACE inhibitors
Angiotensin II receptor blockers
Oral nitrates and hydralazine
Beta blockers
Digoxin
Other inotropes
New drugs in development for heart failure

Treatment objectives

- Increase survival rate
- Decrease morbidity
- Increase exercise capacity
- Improve quality of life
- Decrease neurohormonal changes
- Decelerate progression of CHF
- Reduce symptoms

Together with nonpharmacological measures, diuretics and angiotensin converting enzyme (ACE) inhibitors remain the basis of treatment in patients with congestive heart failure.

In several landmark heart failure studies, the ACE inhibitors have been shown to reduce mortality and to improve symptoms and cardiac parameters. There is now also evidence for beta blockers to be used in chronic stable heart failure, leading to improvements in survival and symptoms. Spironolactone and other aldosterone antagonists may also be beneficial, as indeed are angiotensin II receptor blockers (ARBs), the latter being preferred if ACE inhibitors are not tolerated. Antithrombotic treatment, digoxin and nitrate–hydralazine combination therapy may have possible roles to play in chronic heart failure (Table 7.1).

Newer therapies are being developed to improve treatment and support in acute or severe decompensated heart failure. Drug groups such as the phosphodiesterase inhibitors and calcium sensitizers are far from ready for common use, however.

Diuretics

Although loop and thiazide diuretics have not been shown to improve the outcome in patients with chronic heart failure, they are very effective in providing symptomatic relief. Two types of diuretic are commonly used: loop and thiazide diuretics. These agents are normally

Table 7.1
Pharmacological therapy

	Improved symptoms	Decreased mortality	Prevention of CHF	Neurohormonal control
Diuretics	yes	?	?	no
Digoxin	yes	=	minimal	yes
Inotropes	yes	(increased)	?	no
Nitrates	yes	yes	?	no
ACE inhibitors	yes	yes	yes	yes
Beta blockers	yes	yes	yes	yes
Spironolactone	yes	yes	yes	yes
Other neurohormonal control drugs	yes	+/-	?	yes

first line agents in the treatment of both acute and chronic heart failure, and may be used in combination for an added diuretic effect in fluid retention.

Loop diuretics

Loop diuretics (eg frusemide, bumetanide and torasemide) are powerful diuretics, which inhibit sodium and water reabsorption via their action on the ascending limb of the loop of Henle.

They may cause hyponatraemia and hypokalaemia, and care is needed to avoid hypotension. Long term treatment with high dose diuretics may also cause gout. Frusemide and bumetanide are similar in activity, acting within an hour of oral administration and having effects that last for about six hours. They can therefore be given twice a day without interfering with sleep.

Intravenous administration of frusemide is particularly useful in providing rapid relief of breathlessness and preload in acute pulmonary oedema. Its effects should peak within 30 minutes.

More resistant oedema may require combination therapy with a thiazide (or thiazide-like) diuretic. Bumetanide is useful in the treatment of congestive heart failure when oral absorption of frusemide is reduced.

Thiazide diuretics

Thiazides such as bendrofluazide (bendroflumethiazide) are mild to moderately potent diuretics that inhibit sodium reabsorption at the beginning of the distal convoluted tubule. Like loop diuretics, they act quickly (within 1–2 hours of oral administration) but their effects last for about 12–24 hours. Although their diuretic effects are relatively weak, thiazides are effective antihypertensive agents.

Hyponatraemia and hypokalaemia are commonly associated with higher doses of

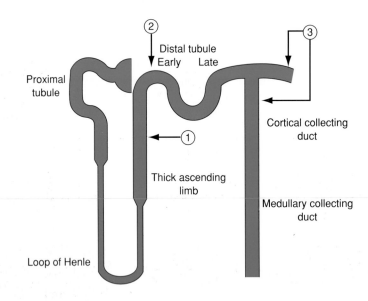

Figure 7.1
Sites and mechanism of action of diuretics in the renal collecting system. 1, 2 and 3 indicate sites of different diuretic class: (1) loop (eg frusemide); (2) thiazide (eg bendrofluazide); (3) potassium sparing (eg amiloride).

thiazide diuretics, and potassium supplementation, or concomitant treatment with a potassium sparing agent, is usually needed with high dose thiazide therapy. Because they have different sites of action, thiazide diuretics may be combined with loop diuretics to produce a greater diuretic effect (Figure 7.1). The thiazide-like agent metolazone is particularly effective as combination therapy with loop diuretics but may cause profound diuresis with electrolyte abnormalities, so any patient on such a regime should be monitored carefully.

Indapamide is a thiazide-like diuretic that lowers blood pressure with less metabolic disturbance and aggravation of diabetes mellitus than bendrofluazide. It has been shown recently that, unlike other thiazide diuretics, it reduces progression of left ventricular hypertrophy in hypertension.

> Loop and thiazide diuretics may be used in combination, but careful monitoring is required

Potassium sparing diuretics

Amiloride and triamterene are weak diuretics that act on the distal nephron. Spironolactone is also a potassium sparing agent, and potentiates thiazide or loop diuretics by antagonizing aldosterone (Figure 7.2). These agents are mainly used when hypokalaemia with the other diuretics is a problem. They should never be given in conjunction with potassium supplements in view of the risk of hyperkalaemia.

A recent study (RALES) suggests that low dose spironolactone (up to 25 mg daily) may be beneficial in severe heart failure in improving morbidity and mortality when used as an adjunct to standard diuretic (eg frusemide) and ACE inhibitor therapy (Figure 7.3). The study also showed that hyperkalaemia is uncommon with this regime, especially if the renal function is normal and the serum biochemistry is monitored. Thus, it is important to measure serum creatinine and potassium concentrations within one week of the addition of a potassium sparing diuretic to an ACE inhibitor until the levels are stable, and then every one to three months.

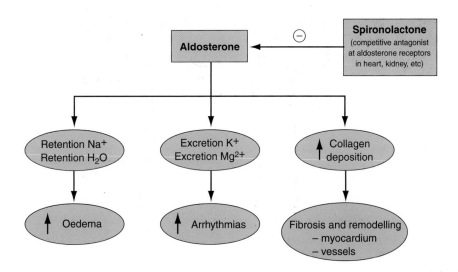

Figure 7.2
Mechanism of action of spironolactone.

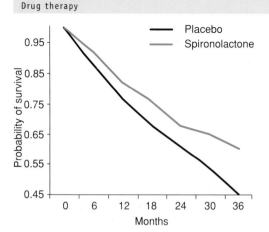

Figure 7.3
RALES study: mortality reduction by 30% among severe heart failure patients (NYHA IV) treated with spironolactone. Adapted from Pitt *et al*, *N Eng J Med* 1999; **341**: 709.

ACE inhibitors

ACE inhibitors (Figure 7.4) have a valuable role to play in all grades of heart failure and, together with diuretics and digoxin when appropriate, form the basis of heart failure treatment. ACE inhibitors have consistently produced beneficial effects on mortality, morbidity and quality of life in large scale prospective clinical trials. Trials such as V-HeFT, CONSENSUS, SOLVD, AIRE, SAVE and TRACE have demonstrated dramatic survival benefits in asymptomatic and symptomatic left ventricular dysfunction and following myocardial infarction, regardless of the presence of symptoms (Table 7.2).

ACE inhibitors are also indicated in hypertension, and are particularly important for hypertension in association with insulin-dependent diabetics with nephropathy.

ACE inhibitors inhibit the conversion of angiotensin I to the metabolically active angiotensin II, a potent vasoconstrictor. As a side effect, bradykinin levels are increased through the inhibition of its degradation. Bradykinin is a vasodilator that has been shown to have beneficial effects associated with the release of nitric oxide and prostacyclin, which may contribute to the positive haemodynamic effects of the ACE inhibitors. Bradykinin may also be responsible, however, for some of the

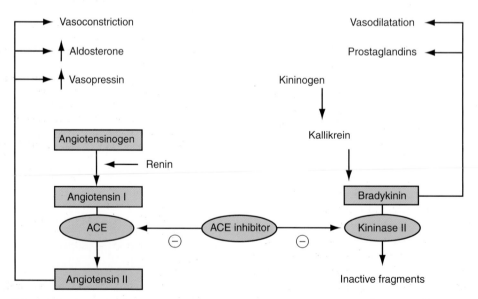

Figure 7.4
Mechanism of action of ACE inhibitors.

Table 7.2

Meta-analysis of effects of ACE inhibitors on mortality and admissions in chronic heart failure

No of trials	Total no of patients	Placebo (%)	Active treatment (%)	Risk reduction (%)	pvalue
32	7105	32.6	22.4	35	<0.001

Adapted from Garg R, Yusuf S. *JAMA* 1995; **273**: 1450–6.

adverse effects, such as dry cough, hypotension and angio-oedema. Other effects of ACE inhibitors are reduction of noradrenaline release and reuptake, upregulation of beta receptor density and improvements in heart rate variability and baroceptor function.

ACE inhibitors should be started at a low dose and gradually titrated to the highest tolerated maintenance level, because of their relative risk of first dose hypotension. ACE inhibitors should be used with particular caution for patients receiving diuretics because of the higher risk of inducing rapid falls in blood pressure. Care and monitoring are also required when used in the presence of peripheral vascular disease or generalized atherosclerosis, owing to the risk of clinically silent renovascular disease (Table 7.3). ACE inhibitors are unlikely to have an adverse effect on renal function in patients with serious unilateral renal artery stenosis but could cause severe and progressive renal failure in patients with bilateral disease, because of their reduction of glomerular filtration. ACE inhibitors are also contraindicated in patients with symptomatic aortic stenosis and outflow tract obstruction. Their side effects include cough, dizziness, deterioration in renal function and (rarely) angio-oedema.

Low-risk patients suitable for home initiation of ACE-I therapy may be started on a small dose of a long-acting ACE inhibitor such as lisinopril 2.5 mg od given at bedtime. Higher-risk patients are best started on short-acting types such as captopril 6.25 mg. Perindopril, which is a long-acting inhibitor, has been shown to carry a lower risk of first dose hypotension and may be used in higher-risk groups as well as low-risk patients. There is some evidence that patients

Table 7.3

Guidelines for using ACE inhibitors

If patient is at high risk of developing complications, initiate first dose at practice surgery, or admit to hospital (see notes below):

- Stop potassium supplements and potassium sparing diuretics
- Omit (or reduce) diuretics for 24 hours before first dose
- Advise patient to sit or lie down for 2–4 hours after first dose. Low-risk patients may take their first dose at home just before going to bed
- Start low doses (for example, captopril 6.25 mg twice daily, enalapril 2.5 mg once daily, lisinopril 2.5 mg once daily)
- Blood pressure should be checked at 2–4 hours for high-risk patients at practice surgery or in hospital
- Review after 1–2 weeks to reassess symptoms, blood pressure, and renal chemistry and electrolytes
- Increase dose unless there has been a rise in serum creatinine concentration (to >200 µmol/litre) or potassium concentration (to >5.0 mmol/litre)
- Titrate to maximum tolerated dose, reassessing blood pressure and renal chemistry and electrolytes after each dose titration
- Aim for doses used in the major trials: captopril 25–50 mg tds; enalapril 10 mg bd; lisinopril 10–20 mg od; ramipril 5 mg bd; trandolapril 4 mg od

High-risk patients requiring supervision at practice surgery or hospital admission to start ACE inhibitor:

- Severe heart failure (NYHA class IV) or decompensated heart failure
- Low systolic blood pressure (<100 mmHg)
- Resting tachycardia >100 beats/min
- Low serum sodium concentration (<130 mmol/litre)
- Other vasodilator treatment
- Severe chronic obstructive airways disease and pulmonary heart disease (cor pulmonale)

with heart failure maintained on higher doses of ACE inhibitors have fewer rehospitalizations than have those on low doses.

> ACE inhibitors have a valuable role to play in all grades of heart failure

Angiotensin II receptor blockers

Orally active angiotensin II type-1 receptor antagonists (Figure 7.5), such as losartan and valsartan, have many properties similar to ACE inhibitors, although their benefit in patients with heart failure has yet to be fully established. They do not inhibit the degradation of bradykinin and other kinins and therefore do not appear to give rise to the persistent cough seen with ACE inhibitor use. Hence they are suitable alternatives for patients not tolerating these side effects of ACE inhibitor therapy.

Larger randomized trials are under way with the aim of determining the effects of angiotensin II receptor antagonists on symptoms and outcome. The studies so far concluded, such as ELITE, ELITE-II and Val-HeFT, have suggested that ARBs appear to be better tolerated and perhaps as good as ACE inhibitors in reducing hospitalizations and mortality. Interestingly, the Val-HeFT trial suggested that combination treatment with an ACE inhibitor and valsartan reduced the composite endpoint of 'death and rehospitalization' by a third, although the effect was less impressive among patients taking beta blockers (Table 7.4). In patients intolerant of ACE inhibitors, valsartan was superior to placebo in reducing endpoints.

Oral nitrates and hydralazine

Oral nitrates can be considered in any patients with ischaemic heart disease and

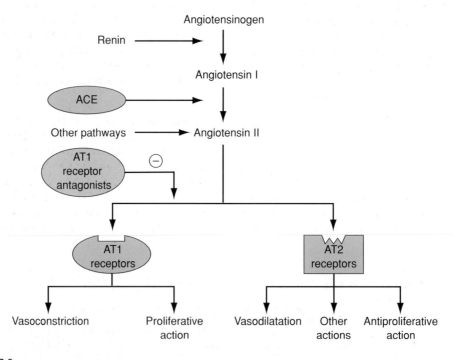

Figure 7.5
Mechanism of action of angiotensin II inhibitors.

Table 7.4
Reduction in total deaths and cardiovascular hospitalizations with addition of valsartan to standard therapy

Variable	Events		Relative risk (CI)	pvalue
	Vasartan n=2511	Placebo n=2499		
All-cause mortality	495 (19.7%)	484 (19.4%)	1.02 (0.90, 1.15)	0.800
Combined all-cause mortality + morbidity	723 (28.8%)	801 (32.1%)	0.87 (0.79, 0.96)	0.009

Data presented at the American Heart Association Meeting (November 2000)

impaired left ventricular systolic function. A nitrate-free period of between four and eight hours prevents the development of tolerance in patients on long-acting nitrate preparations.

Hydralazine has been shown to improve survival in patients with mild to moderate heart failure when used in combination with nitrates (Figure 7.7), although the survival rates are still better with ACE inhibitors. The combination of nitrates and hydralazine is thus a useful alternative for patients who cannot tolerate ACE inhibitors or ARBs (as in severe renal impairment). There is some evidence that a nitrate–hydralazine combination may be more effective in black patients with hypertension who develop heart failure.

Beta blockers

Previously contraindicated in heart failure for a perceived fear of their negative inotropy, recent evidence has now firmly established the benefit of beta-adrenoceptor antagonists (or beta blockers) in chronic heart failure.

Clinical studies using the second generation beta-1 selective bisoprolol and metoprolol, and the third generation nonselective carvedilol with vasodilatory alpha-blocking actions, have shown a dramatic improvement to symptoms, exercise tolerance, left ventricular function and survival when these agents are added to conventional treatment. The mortality reduction in these studies (CIBIS II, MERIT-HF, combined US carvedilol, ANZ, COPERNICUS) ranged between 30 and 60%, with benefit evident in all patient groups with NYHA classes II to IV (Table 7.5).

Beta blockers should be initiated cautiously, starting at very low doses, and can be titrated to maximum tolerated doses *very slowly* over a period of two or three months ('go slow, go low'). They should not be started within six weeks of acute decompensated heart failure. Patients should be observed for side effects of vasodilatation (such as dizziness and light-

Table 7.5
Meta-analysis of effects of beta blockers on mortality and admissions to hospital in chronic heart failure

No of trials	Total no of patients	Placebo (%)	Active treatment (%)	Risk reduction (%)	pvalue
18	3023	24.6	15.8	38	<0.001

Adapted from Lechat P, Packer M, Chalon S *et al. Circulation* 1998; **98**: 1184–91.

headedness) for the first 2–4 hours and continue to be reviewed for features of worsening heart failure during the period of titration (Table 7.6).

> The benefit of beta blockers in chronic heart failure has been firmly established

Digoxin

Digoxin, a cardiac glycoside, is a positive inotrope and also reduces conductivity within the atrioventricular node. It is potentially most useful when used in patients with atrial fibrillation and coexistent heart failure, in whom it can improve control of the ventricular rate to allow for more effective filling of the ventricle. Beyond that the role of digoxin is less clear, particularly for chronic heart failure in sinus rhythm. (For the mechanism of action of digoxin, see Figure 7.8.)

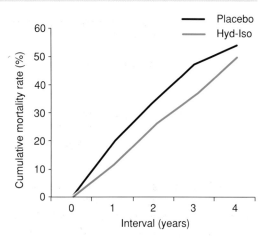

Figure 7.7
V-HeFT study: Addition of hydralazine nitrate (Hyd-Iso) to digoxin and diuretics in the treatment of congestive heart failure reduces mortality by 25%. Adapted from Cohn J, Archibald D, Ziesche S *et al. N Engl J Med* 1986; **314**: 1547–52.

Table 7.6
Titration schedule for carvedilol and bisoprolol according to manufacturer's instructions

Patients should not have any symptoms of worsening heart failure, bradycardia (<50/min), hypotension (<90 mmHg) or persistent symptoms of vasodilatation (dizziness) before titrating up to the next dose. If these features are present, the drug should be maintained at the same dose, reduced or withdrawn

Carvedilol		*Bisoprolol*
Start at 3.125 mg bd for at least two weeks	Initiation and Week 1 Week 2	Start at 1.25 mg od 2.5 mg od
Then 6.25 mg bd for at least two weeks	Week 3 Week 4	3.75 mg od Then 5 mg od for four weeks
Then 12.5 mg bd for at least two weeks	Week 5 Week 6	
Then 25 mg bd (maximum maintenance dose if patient weight <85 kg)	Week 7 Week 8	Then 7.5 mg od for four weeks
If patient weight >85 kg, increase to 50 mg bd (maximum maintenance dose)	Week 9 Week 10 Week 11 Week 12	Then 10 mg od (maximum maintenance dose)

Beta blockers in congestive cardiac failure	
Who benefits?	NYHA II–IV
	Full conventional Rx
What are the benefits?	Improved survival
	Reduced hospitalizations
	Long term symptom improvement
	Decreased transplantation
What are the costs?	Early symptomatic deterioration
'Go low, go slow...'	

Several trials have shown that discontinuing digoxin in patients with chronic heart failure leads to increased hospitalization. The Digitalis Investigation Group (DIG) found that digoxin further improves heart failure symptoms when added to diuretics and ACE inhibitors (Figure 7.9). There was no overall reduction in mortality, however, and there was even a small trend towards an excess where arrhythmic complications were present.

Digoxin can therefore be considered for patients with sinus rhythm who remain symptomatic despite optimal doses of diuretics and ACE inhibitors. It may also be useful in cases of severe left ventricular systolic dysfunction and dilatation where it acts as an inotrope, or where there have been recurrent hospital admissions for heart failure.

> Increased admissions to hospital have been recorded in patients with chronic heart failure when digoxin administration has been discontinued

Digoxin has a long half-life. For patients with mild heart failure, a loading dose is not usually required, and a satisfactory plasma concentration can be achieved with a dose of 250 µg daily for a week, which is then reduced, if needed.

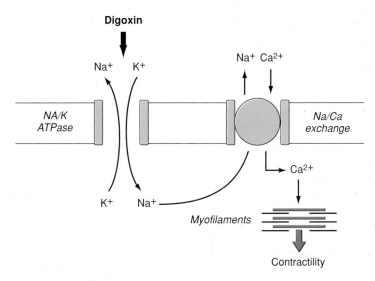

Figure 7.8
Mechanism of action of digoxin.

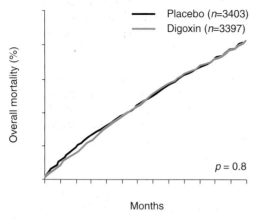

Figure 7.9
Reduction of death or hospitalization for worsening heart failure when digoxin is added to diuretics and ACE inhibitors. Adapted from the Digitalis Investigation Group. *N Engl J Med* 1997; **336**: 525–33.

Toxicity can be exacerbated by hypokalaemia and therefore potassium levels should be checked before initiation of therapy, especially when added to nonpotassium sparing diuretics.

> Digoxin is the only positive inotrope that is valuable in the management of chronic heart failure

Other inotropes

Newer inotropes are being evaluated for heart failure. To date, none of the inotropes improve the dreadful prognosis in heart failure; in decompensated patients inotropes may even increase mortality, albeit at some symptomatic benefit.

The bipyridine phosphodiesterase III (PDE-III) inhibitors (eg vesnarinone, milrinone, enoximone and amrinone) form a new class of positive inotropic vasodilator agents in the treatment of acute and chronic heart failure. They increase levels of intracellular cyclic adenosine monophosphate (cAMP) by inhibiting its intracellular hydrolysis, which results in greater myocardial contractility plus peripheral vasodilatation. Clinical trials have shown short

term intermittent infusion with milrinone to be safe, efficacious and cost-effective and milrinone is now approved for use as intravenous administration in the treatment of decompensated congestive heart failure. Other phosphodiesterase III inhibitors have similarly demonstrated beneficial short term effects, although longer term treatment has been associated with increased mortality from sudden cardiac deaths.

A new agent, levosimendan, which is a calcium sensitizer inotrope, appears to have some beneficial effect in decompensated heart failure, even in patients with myocardial infarction, with no excess mortality in recent small trials. Further information is awaited with interest.

For now, digoxin remains the only positive inotrope (albeit a weak one) that is valuable in the management of chronic heart failure.

New drugs in development for heart failure

Analogues of natriuretic peptides and medicines that modulate endothelin and cytokine release and endothelial vasoconstriction are being developed and may well prove to useful in the future management of heart failure.

Nesiritide is a human B-type natriuretic peptide analogue that has been shown to provide beneficial haemodynamic effects when used as a first line intravenous agent in patients with acute decompensated heart failure. ANP is broken down by the enzyme neural endopeptidase (NEP), and drugs that inhibit this enzyme (such as candoxatril) therefore increase the availability of natriuretic peptides. Its clinical benefits are still being evaluated.

Bosentan is a specific endothelin-1 receptor antagonist. It is the first agent in this group of drugs to enter phase III clinical trials and the results so far have been promising. Bosentan may also regulate coronary vascular tone and might prove to be useful in coronary artery disease, which often coexists with heart failure. Long term studies are still needed to elucidate its modes of action and objective benefit.

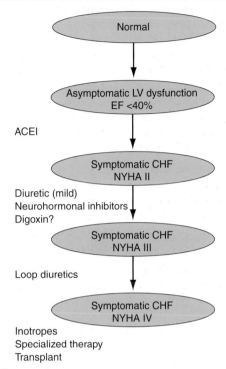

Figure 7.10
Heart failure treatment summary.

Antithrombotic treatment

Patients with chronic heart failure have an increased risk of stroke and thromboembolism. This risk is significantly higher in the presence of atrial and left ventricular dilatation, left ventricular aneurysm or mural thrombus formation, atrial fibrillation and previous stroke history.

Patients with heart failure in atrial fibrillation require anticoagulation with warfarin. It still remains to be seen if anticoagulation is warranted for heart failure patients in sinus rhythm. Although many trials have suggested the benefit of warfarin in stroke prevention, most of these trials were small, nonrandomized and retrospective in nature. On-going large clinical studies such as WATCH (Warfarin Antiplatelet Therapy in Chronic Heart Failure) will eventually determine the safety and efficacy of anticoagulation for

heart failure, compared with antiplatelet therapy. This question is pertinent, as there appears to be some suggestion that an interaction between aspirin and the ACE inhibitors may actually reduce the efficacy of the latter agents. Furthermore, the data indicating that aspirin convincingly reduces mortality in heart failure *per se* are limited, while it is clear that aspirin can increase the risk of gastrointestinal problems and bleeding.

Currently, consideration should be given to starting anticoagulation in patients with idiopathic dilated cardiomyopathy, severe systolic impairment in the presence of mobile, protruding left ventricular mural thrombus, in the setting of left ventricular aneurysm after extensive myocardial infarction, and in those with a history of previous stroke.

Antiarrhythmic treatment

Amiodarone is useful in the treatment of ventricular and supraventricular arrhythmias, including atrial fibrillation. With atrial fibrillation of recent onset, treatment with amiodarone increases the long term success rate of cardioversion. Amiodarone is also effective in controlling ventricular arrhythmias in chronic heart failure.

Class I antiarrhythmic agents are associated with increased mortality in heart failure and are therefore contraindicated. Digoxin can be used in chronic atrial fibrillation for ventricular rate control.

In recurrent ventricular arrhythmias associated with left ventricular impairment, some consideration should be given towards use of an implantable cardioverter–defibrillator, in addition to amiodarone.

Further reading

Australia/New Zealand Heart Failure Research Collaborative Group. Randomized, placebo-controlled trial of carvedilol in patients with congestive heart failure due to ischaemic heart disease. *Lancet* 1997; **349**: 375–80.

Cohn JN, Archibald DG, Ziesche S *et al.* Effect of vasodilator therapy on mortality in chronic congestive heart failure. Results of a Veterans Administraiton Cooperative Study. *N Engl J Med* 1986; **314**: 1547–52.

CONSENSUS Trial Study Group. Effects of enalapril on mortality in severe congestive heart failure: results of the cooperative north Scandinavian enalapril survival study (CONSENSUS). *N Engl J Med* 1987; **316**: 1429–35.

Digitalis Investigation Group. The effect of digoxin on mortality and morbidity in patients with heart failure. *N Engl J Med* 1997; **336**: 525–33.

Doval HC, Nul DR, Grancelli HO *et al.* Randomised trial of low dose amiodarone in severe congestive heart failure (GESICA trial). *Lancet* 1994; **344**: 493–8.

Harjai KJ, Nunez E, Turgut T, Newman J. Effect of combined aspirin and angiotensin-converting enzyme inhibitor therapy versus angiotensin-converting enzyme inhibitor therapy alone on readmission rates in heart failure. *Am J Cardiol* 2001; **87**: 483–7.

Lip GYH, Gibbs CR. Anticoagulation for heart failure in sinus rhythm (Cochrane Review). In: *Cochrane Library*, Issue 4. Oxford: Update Software, 2001.

Lip GYH, Gibbs CR. Antiplatelet agents versus control or anticoagulation for heart failure in sinus rhythm (Cochrane Review). In: *Cochrane Library*, Issue 4. Oxford: Update Software, 2001

MERIT-HF Study Group. Effect of metoprolol CR/XL in chronic heart failure: metoprolol CR/XL randomised intervention trial in congestive heart failure (MERIT-HF). *Lancet* 1999; **353**: 2001–7.

Packer M, Bristow MR, Cohn JN *et al.* Effect of carvedilol on morbidity and mortality in patients with chronic heart failure. *N Engl J Med* 1996; **334**: 1349–55.

Pitt B, Zannad F, Remme WJ *et al.* The effect of spironolactone on morbidity and mortality in patients with severe heart failure. *N Engl J Med* 1999; **314**: 709–71.

SOLVD Investigators. Effect of enalapril on mortality and the development of heart failure in asymptomatic patients with reduced left ventricular ejection fractions. *N Engl J Med* 1992; **327**: 685–91.

8. Management pathways for heart failure

Management of acute heart failure
Management of chronic heart failure
Treatment of underlying disease
Cardiac transplantation
Heart failure management in general practice
Conclusion

Management of both acute and chronic heart failure is aimed at alleviating symptoms, removing or treating the underlying cause and improving survival.

Management of acute heart failure

Assessment

Patients with acute heart failure commonly complain of orthopnoea or paroxysmal nocturnal dyspnoea (Table 8.1). They may present with dyspnoea at rest, tachycardia and, in more severe cases, pallor and hypotension.

Cardiogenic shock is diagnosed when there is hypotension, oliguria and low cardiac output. It can occur following extensive myocardial infarction, acute rupture of papillary muscle or sustained arrhythmias.

Treatment (see Table 8.2)

The patient should be nursed sitting in an upright position with high concentration oxygen (6–10 litres/min) delivered via a face mask. Sublingual glyceryl nitrate, in a dose of 0.5–2 mg, is quick and easy to administer.

Once peripheral intravenous access has been established, intravenous loop diuretics (such as

Table 8.1
Clinical features of patients in acute and chronic heart failure

Acute heart failure
- Distressed, dyspnoeic
- Cold clammy skin, pallor (features of poor perfusion)
- Hypotension (systolic <90 mmHg)
- Tachycardia (>100/min)
- Displaced and forceful apex beat
- Right ventricular heave
- Third and/or fourth heart sounds – gallop rhythm can be heard if accompanying tachycardia
- Murmur of functional mitral or tricuspid regurgitation
- Fluid retention: raised JVP, lung crepitations, liver congestion, peripheral oedema

Chronic heart failure
- May include all of the above depending on degree of compensation, plus:
- Skeletal muscle wasting (cardiac cachexia)
- Cheyne–Stokes respiratory pattern

Other features that may indicate underlying aetiology
- Murmur of aortic stenosis or other primary valvular disease
- General atherosclerotic disease
- Hypertension
- Anaemia or volume overload
- Haemodynamically important arrhythmia
- Systemic diseases

frusemide 80 mg or bumetanide 2 mg) should be given together with intravenous diamorphine 2.5–5 mg. Loop diuretics given intravenously act quickly and induce transient venodilatation even before the onset of diuresis, and are thus helpful in providing rapid relief of symptoms.

Intravenous opiates also induce venodilatation but are important too in relieving pain, anxiety and distress, thus reducing myocardial oxygen demand. Intravenous nitrate infusion is helpful in further reducing preload and is particularly useful for patients with coexisting anginal chest pains, high blood pressure or continuing pulmonary congestion. A further bolus of loop diuretic can be administered after 30 minutes if the patient remains symptomatic and is not hypotensive.

Table 8.2
Management of acute heart failure

Basic measures and initial drug treatment:
- Sit patient upright
- Give oxygen 35–60%
- Attach an ECG monitor and treat arrhythmias
- Frusemide 40–80 mg IV
- Diamorphine 2.5–5 mg IV slowly (plus anti-emetic cover)
- If systolic BP >90 mmHg, give nitrate sublingually (GTN two puffs) or buccally (2–5 mg)
- Urgent investigations: ECG, chest X-ray, arterial blood gases, biochemistry and, if cause of acute heart failure in doubt, echocardiogram
- Recheck BP in 20 minutes

Second line drug treatment and advanced management:
- If systolic BP >100 mmHg,
  - give further frusemide 40–80 mg IV
  - start a nitrate infusion, increasing infusion rate every 15–30 min to alleviate breathlessness but keeping BP ~100 mmHg
  - patients with renal failure may require frusemide infusion; if this fails, arrange for dialysis
- If systolic BP 80–100 mmHg,
  - start dobutamine infusion at 5 µg/kg/min and increase every 10 min until BP >100 mmHg (maximum 20 µg/kg/min)
  - add nitrate infusion if needed, once BP >100 mmHg
- If systolic BP < 80 mmHg (cardiogenic shock),
  - start dobutamine infusion at 5 µg/kg/min and increase every 10 min until BP >100 mmHg (maximum 20 µg/kg/min)
  - start a dopamine infusion at 10 µg/kg/min via a central venous line and titrate up to 20 µg/kg/min (low dose dopamine has not been shown to improve or preserve renal function)
- If BP still <90 mmHg despite maximum dopamine dose, change over to noradrenaline 0.05–5 µg/kg/min
- Consider phosphodiesterase inhibitors such as enoximone
- Consider:
  - Swan–Ganz catheterization, aiming for pulmonary artery wedge pressure of 15–20 mmHg
  - assisted ventilation if pO_2 <8 kPa despite 60% oxygen, or if pCO_2 is rising
  - ventricular assist devices if corrective surgery (valvular or septal defect) is planned or where a chance of spontaneous recovery exists (eg peripartum cardiomyopathy)

Frequent monitoring of pulse, blood pressure and urinary output are required in the early hours of treatment. Basic investigations are essential, and should include chest X-ray, 12-lead electrocardiograph and examination of venous blood samples at the biochemistry and haematology labs. Arterial blood gases provide valuable information about oxygenation and acid–base balance. The 'base excess' is a guide to actual tissue perfusion in patients with acute heart failure; increasingly negative base excess indicates worsening lactic acidosis secondary to increasing dependency upon anaerobic metabolism, and is an indicator of poor prognosis. Correction of hypoperfusion will correct the metabolic acidosis; bicarbonate infusions should be reserved for the most refractory cases.

Any underlying cause of acute heart failure should be corrected. Rhythm disturbances are frequent but do not always require treatment. Complete heart block following acute myocardial infarction may require temporary pacing, in the setting of haemodynamic compromise. Sinus bradycardia and first-degree block can often remain untreated if not associated with haemodynamic instability. Atropine (600 µg intravenously) can be used in symptomatic bradycardia in inferior myocardial infarction to overcome high vagal stimulation.

Sinus tachycardias are often present and are caused by pain and anxiety. Persistent tachycardias may indicate extensive cardiac muscle loss and are associated with poorer prognosis. Gentle intravenous beta blockade (metoprolol 2–5 mg slowly) may be tried with great caution.

> Intravenous opiates are important in relieving pain, anxiety and distress

Sustained tachyarrhythmias should be corrected quickly, on account of the increased myocardial demand placed upon the myocardium. Supraventricular tachycardia may be abolished with intravenous adenosine. The development of atrial fibrillation is usually in the setting of large infarcts and may indicate significant cardiac dysfunction. In most cases, atrial fibrillation is transient and self-limiting; cardioversion is not necessarily needed unless haemodynamic compromise occurs. Nevertheless intravenous (unfractionated) heparin or subcutaneous low-molecular-weight heparin should be commenced to minimize the risk of thromboembolism.

The development of ventricular arrhythmias in the acute setting of an infarct does not necessarily demand long term prophylaxis, although the development of recurrent ventricular arrhythmias remote from the time of infarction (for example, 'secondary' ventricular tachycardia) may require further assessment and treatment. Consultation with a cardiac electrophysiologist may be helpful.

Intravenous amiodarone may be used for both supraventricular and ventricular arrhythmias, and finally electrical cardioversion is indicated if urgent restoration of sinus rhythm is required (as in cardiogenic shock).

Short term inotropic support

Cardiogenic shock and severe refractory heart failure in which the cardiac output remains critically low require agents with positive inotropic properties such as the sympathomimetic agents (dobutamine, dopamine and adrenaline) and phosphodiesterase inhibitors. Inotropic agents in general increase the potential for cardiac arrhythmias.

Vasoconstrictor sympathomimetics act on alpha-adrenergic receptors to cause peripheral vasoconstriction. Thus blood pressure is raised at the expense of perfusion to vital organs such as the kidney. They usually also act on alpha and beta receptors in the heart to increase heart rate and contractility. They are therefore not suitable for use in myocardial infarction and ischaemic heart disease but are useful in septic shock.

Cardiac stimulants such as dobutamine act on beta-1 receptors in cardiac muscle and are positively inotropic without increasing heart rate. Dobutamine may therefore be useful in cardiogenic shock following extensive myocardial infarction. The dose of dopamine infusion is critical because at low concentrations dopamine acts as a vasodilator and increases renal perfusion, but at higher levels (>5 µg/kg/min) it induces vasoconstriction and may even exacerbate heart failure. Recent evidence suggests that the so-called 'renal dose dopamine' is no better than placebo in renoprotection, and may even increase the risk of arrhythmias. Thus, renal dose dopamine should be avoided in heart failure.

> Dopamine may act as either a vasoconstrictor or a vasodilator, according to dosage

Dopexamine acts on beta-2 receptors in cardiac muscle and peripherally to increase renal perfusion without vasoconstriction. The newer phosphodiesterase inhibitors (for example, enoximone) are established for short term use as intravenous infusions in severe heart failure. Long term use of these agents is associated with increased mortality.

Intravenous aminophylline is now rarely used for treating acute heart failure.

Intra-aortic balloon pumping and mechanical devices

Patients with acute heart failure requiring support may benefit from short term use of ventricular assist devices. Mechanical devices are indicated as a bridge to cardiac surgery (in the case of lesions such as ruptured papillary muscle or ventricular septal defect postmyocardial infarction) or transplantation or when there is a possibility of spontaneous recovery (for example, peripartum cardiomyopathy, myocarditis) in severe heart failure. Intra-aortic balloon counterpulsation is the most commonly used form of mechanical support.

Management of chronic heart failure

The objectives of chronic heart failure management are control of symptoms, reduction of hospitalizations and the improvement of survival.

> Loop diuretics and ACE inhibitors are the mainstay of therapy for chronic heart failure

For many patients whose heart failure is stable and compensated, there may be few or no symptoms or clinical features. Patients with chronic heart failure may become decompensated. Such patients normally present acutely with dypsnoea at rest, pulmonary

oedema and fluid retention, or more gradually with deteriorating exercise tolerance, increasing dypsnoea, lethargy and lower limb oedema. The cause or causes of decompensation should be identified. Common precipitants are rapid atrial fibrillation, infection, recurrent ischaemia, electrolyte disturbance and drug noncompliance (Table 8.4). Patients with acute decompensation may need admission to hospital for treatment as with acute heart failure.

Overcoming fluid overload may be difficult despite large doses of loop diuretics. Such patients with severe congestive heart failure may require additional diuretics, or combination diuretic therapy with metolazone or bendrofluazide, along with fluid restriction to 1–1.5 litres per day. Salt restriction may also be beneficial. The patient should be weighed daily to monitor fluid loss and response to diuretics.

Patients with more gradual deterioration or whose heart dysfunction is stable and compensated can be managed in the outpatients department. As well as pharmacological treatment, patients should also be offered advice and counselling on lifestyle changes, diet and exercise.

Loop diuretics and ACE inhibitors are the mainstay of therapy for chronic heart failure. Patients not tolerating ACE inhibitors because of cough or other ACE-I specific side effects may be tried on an angiotensin II receptor blocker. Patients who are stable can be given beta blockers (carvedilol, bisoprolol, metoprolol) but require low dose initiation and

Table 8.3
Management of chronic heart failure

- *General:*
  - Counselling and support
  - Advice on diet, exercise and maintaining optimal weight
  - Stop smoking and restrict alcohol intake
  - Treat cardiovascular risk factors (hyperlipidaemia, diabetes mellitus) and hypertension
  - Asymptomatic left ventricular dysfunction (NYHA I)
  - ACE inhibitor
- *Mild heart failure (NYHA II):*
  - ACE inhibitor
  - Thiazide or loop diuretics
  - Consider beta blockers
- *Moderate heart failure (NYHA II–III):*
  - ACE inhibitor
  - Loop diuretic
  - Beta blocker
- *Severe heart failure (NYHA IV):*
  - ACE inhibitor
  - Increase loop diuretic to overcome fluid overload
  - Add a thiazide diuretic (eg metolazone) if necessary
  - Consider spironolactone, beta blockers and antithrombotic therapy
- *End-stage intractable heart failure:*
  - As for severe heart failure
  - Consider cardiac transplantation, cardiomyoplasty

Table 8.4
Causes of readmission in patients with heart failure

- Angina
- Infections
- Arrhythmias
- Poor compliance or inadequate drug treatment
- Iatrogenic factors, eg worsening heart failure following initiation of beta blocker therapy
- Inadequate discharge planning or follow-up
- Poor social support

cautious titration under specialist supervision. Spironolactone is also helpful, but care and frequent biochemical checks are needed when it is added to ACE inhibitor therapy.

Oral digoxin has a role in patients with left ventricular systolic impairment, in sinus rhythm, who remain symptomatic despite optimal doses of diuretics and ACE inhibitors. Warfarin should be considered in patients with atrial fibrillation or severe dilated cardiomyopathy and those who have had previous strokes.

Treatment of underlying disease

Any reversible or treatable causes of heart failure should be managed accordingly to reduce or halt progression of heart failure.

Secondary prevention of ischaemic heart disease is important. Percutaneous coronary angioplasty (PTCA) and coronary artery bypass grafting (CABG) should be offered for patients who would benefit from revascularization. This would clearly include patients with ischaemic heart disease and evidence of hibernating myocardium where revascularization might improve overall left ventricular function.

Good blood pressure control is essential for patients with hypertension. In patients with documented left ventricular hypertrophy or systolic dysfunction, ACE inhibitors are the drugs of choice in view of their benefits in regression of hypertrophy and improving mortality. Hypertension in patients with isolated diastolic dysfunction may be controlled using beta blockers or nondihydropyridine calcium channel blockers.

Valve replacement or repair should be considered for any patients with haemodynamically important primary valvular disease. Impaired ventricular function in itself is not an absolute contraindication to cardiac surgery, although the operative risks are increased.

Patients with resistant ventricular arrhythmias or bradycardias with haemodynamic instability should receive an implantable defibrillator or permanent pacemaker respectively.

Cardiac transplantation

Cardiac transplantation is indicated for patients with end-stage heart failure who are expected to have less than one year to live (one year survival <50%), do not have any other life-limiting or severe systemic illnesses (such as malignancy) and have good social and home support (Table 8.5).

Improvements and experience have reduced perioperative mortality to less than 10%, with one-, five- and ten-year survival now at 90%, 75% and 60%, respectively. Rejection of the transplant is less of a problem with the advent of cyclosporin and other immunosuppressants but can lead to accelerated graft atherosclerosis. The major problem, however, remains the shortage of organ donors; about 25% of patients on the waiting list die before a donor can be found for them. One option may be the use of left ventricular devices as a 'bridge' to transplantation.

Table 8.5
Indications and contraindications to cardiac transplantation in adults

- *Indications:*
  - End-stage heart failure – for example, ischaemic heart disease and dilated cardiomyopathy
  - Rarely, restrictive cardiomyopathy and peripartum cardiomyopathy
  - Congenital heart disease (often combined heart–lung transplantation required)
- *Absolute contraindications:*
  - Recent malignancy (other than basal cell and squamous cell carcinoma of the skin)
  - Active infection (including HIV, hepatitis B, hepatitis C with liver disease)
  - Systemic disease that is likely to affect life expectancy
  - Significant pulmonary vascular resistance
- *Relative contraindications:*
  - Recent pulmonary embolism
  - Symptomatic peripheral vascular disease
  - Obesity
  - Severe renal impairment
  - Psychosocial problems – for example, lack of social support, poor compliance, psychiatric illness
  - Age (over 60–65 years)

Heart failure management in general practice

Medical advances and resource streamlining have combined to make the management of heart failure in general practice more important now than ever before. The prevalence and incidence of patients with heart failure are rising every year. Heart failure treatment is also improving outcome and reducing the need for hospitalization. These factors, coupled with the recent closures of hospital beds, mean that general practitioners are likely to become increasingly involved in the identification, investigation and chronic management of patients with heart failure.

Identifying heart failure in general practice

Heart failure is difficult to diagnose and ventricular dysfunction may not be clinically evident even to the cardiologist. Several studies in the UK and Europe have found that fewer than a third of patients thought to have heart failure by their general practitioners meet the clinical criteria approved by the European Society of Cardiology (see chapter 4).

Access to use of non-invasive investigations such as 12-lead electrocardiography, chest X-ray and echocardiography is important for more accurate diagnoses of heart failure. While it is fairly easy to obtain the first two investigations, direct access to echocardiography is still limited. The reason for this is often said to originate in financial and staffing issues. This may be misleading, however, since the cost of echocardiography (about £50–£70 per person) is far less than the cost of hospitalization and acute treatment would have been in the absence of an early diagnosis of heart failure and the institution of appropriate therapy. Performing a baseline ECG and chest X-ray and referring only those patients with abnormal findings would make it cost beneficial and a good compromise.

Natriuretic peptides have emerged recently as offering a possible practical bedside diagnostic test for heart failure. Plasma concentrations of both atrial natriuretic peptides (ANP) and B-type natriuretic peptide (BNP) are markedly elevated in heart failure and correlate well with severity of left ventricular impairment. In addition, BNP may have up to 97% sensitivity and 84% specificity in identifying heart failure, giving a positive predictive value of about 70%. Given the difficulties in diagnosing heart failure on clinical grounds alone, and the current limitations on open access echocardiography service, plasma BNP measurements make for very attractive diagnostic tools of heart failure in general practice. However, more data are still required.

Primary prevention and progression to heart failure

In addition to identifying heart failure early, GPs also play a vital role in preventing heart failure. In the UK and most developed countries, hypertension and ischaemic heart disease are the main causes of heart failure. A way of stemming the rising incidence of heart failure would be to treat these diseases and their predisposing factors.

Thus patients should be advised to maintain a low-salt, low-fat diet along with plenty of exercise, and to stop smoking. Blood pressure should be observed and treated if it is high. Patients with hyperlipidaemia should be given a statin if appropriate. Secondary prevention in ischaemic heart disease, such as aspirin or beta blockers, should reduce future ischaemic cardiac events.

Patients with left ventricular dysfunction without clinical features or symptoms (asymptomatic ventricular dysfunction) would also benefit from early treatment with ACE inhibitors to minimize the progression to symptomatic heart failure.

> Hypertension and ischaemic heart disease are the main causes of heart failure in the UK

Starting treatment in general practice

Most heart failure drugs can now be started outside hospital. Patients at high risk of complications who may require hospitalization to initiate ACE inhibitors are those with severe or decompensated heart failure, systolic blood pressure less than 100 mmHg, resting tachycardia, low serum sodium concentration (<130 mmol/litre) or using concurrent vasodilators.

Patients with mild or moderate heart failure who have normal renal function and a systolic blood pressure over 100 mmHg are unlikely to have problems if they stop taking their diuretics 24 hours earlier and take their first ACE inhibitor dose at night.

Beta blockers should only be initiated in patients with chronic stable heart failure, with the dose titrated slowly over a period of 2–3 months. Currently, we recommend that beta blockers be initiated at specialist cardiology clinics and that care is shared between the specialist and the general practitioner for observation and titration to the maximum tolerated dose.

Heart failure clinics

General practitioners may set up their own heart failure clinics, attended by a practice nurse with special interest in the subject to manage and monitor these patients. The role of the clinic can include patient education and counselling, review of medications to ensure compliance and adequacy of treatment, monitoring of symptoms and response to therapy as well as to side effects arising from treatments. Cardiovascular risk factors may also be controlled and routine blood chemistry can be sent from the clinic at least every 12 months. Patients who are refractory to conventional treatment or deteriorating should be referred for specialist opinion (Table 8.6).

Specialist nurse support

Specialist nurse support for heart failure has been limited in Britain compared with other

Table 8.6
Conditions indicating that referral to a specialist is necessary

- Diagnosis of heart failure or underlying aetiology in doubt or when specialist investigation and management may help
- Intractable or severe symptom-limited heart failure in a young patient (<65 years) where cardiac transplantation may be an option
- Significant murmurs and valvular heart disease, indicating possible valvular repair or surgery
- Arrhythmias requiring specific drug therapy, pacemaker or implantable defibrillator
- Recurrent ischaemia or evidence of hibernating myocardium where revascularization may be beneficial
- High-risk patients in whom ACE inhibitor initiation in hospital is preferred
- Eligibility to participate in clinical trials or new therapies
- Severe left ventricular impairment eg ejection fraction <20% where closer supervision and multidisciplinary approach may be warranted
- Patients with multiple admissions with heart failure
- Poor response to standard treatment

countries such as the United States and Australia. In both these countries, studies have shown the intervention of specialist nurse support as part of a multidisciplinary approach resulted in a reduction in hospitalizations. Quality of life scores also improved in the intervention group; a 20% mortality reduction was found in the Adelaide (Australia) study, although the study cohort was relatively small.

Conclusion

The message nevertheless is clear: the improved management of heart failure necessitates a multidisciplinary approach, with close liaison between general practitioner, hospital specialist, specialist nurse, dietician, clinical psychologist, etc. Hospital heart failure clinics should facilitate urgent assessment of referrals, including the availability of echocardiography to document the severity of left ventricular dysfunction. These specialist clinics would also enable the supervised initiation of therapy, including ACE inhibitors, as well as optimization of drug treatment, including the up-titration of beta blockers, in view of the marked benefits of this class of drugs in the treatment of patients with heart failure.

Further reading

Remme WJ. The treatment of heart failure. The Task Force of the Working Group on Heart Failure of the European Society of Cardiology. *Eur Heart J* 1997; **18**: 736–53.

Rich MW, Beckham V, Wittenberg C *et al*. A multidisciplinary intervention to prevent the readmission of elderly patients with congestive heart failure. *N Engl J Med* 1995: **333**: 1190–5.

Stewart S, Vandenbroek AJ, Pearson S, Horowitz JD. Prolonged beneficial effects of home-based intervention on unplanned readmissions and mortality among patients with congestive heart failure. *Arch Intern Med* 1999; **159**: 257–61.

Further recommended reading

Gibbs CR, Davies MK, Lip GYH, eds. *ABC of Heart Failure*. London: BMJ Books, 2000.

British National Formulary. London: Royal Pharmaceutical Society of Great Britain and British Medical Association, 2000.

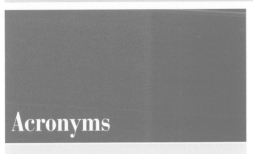

Acronyms

Research studies
Other

Research studies

AIRE	Acute Infarction Ramipril Efficacy (AIRE) Study
ANZ	Australia–New Zealand Heart Failure Research Collaborative Group
CIBIS	Cardiac Insufficiency Bisoprolol Study
CONSENSUS	Cooperative New Scandinavian Enalapril Survival Study
COPERNICUS	Carvedilol Prospective Randomised Cumulative Survival Trial
ECHOES	Echocardiographic Heart of England Screening study
ELITE	Evaluation of Losartan in the Elderly
ELITE-II	Losartan Heart Failure Survival Study

MERIT-HF	Metoprolol Controlled-Release Randomised Intervention Trial in Heart Failure
MONICA	Monitoring Trends And Determinants Of Cardiovascular Disease
PRAISE	Prospective Randomized Amlodipine Survival Evaluation
RALES	Randomized Aldactone Evaluation Study
SAVE	Survival and Ventricular Enlargement
SOLVD-P	Studies of Left Ventricular Dysfunction – Prevention arm
SOLVD-T	Studies of Left Ventricular Dysfunction – Treatment arm
TRACE	TRAndolapril Cardiac Evaluation
V-HeFT	Veterans Heart Failure Trial
Val-HeFT	Valsartan Heart Failure Trial
WATCH	Warfarin Antiplatelet Therapy in Heart Failure

Other

ANP	Atrial Natiuretic Peptide
BNP	Brain Natiuretic Peptide
ESC	European Society of Cardiology
MUGA	MultiGated Analysis
NYHA	New York Heart Association
RAAS	Renin Angiotensin Aldosterone System

Appendix I: Primary care heart failure guidelines

Prevention
Building a heart failure register
Clinical assessment
Management following confirmation of diagnosis at the direct access echo service

Prevention

1   Ensure all patients with established occlusive arterial disease (coronary/cerebrovascular/peripheral artery disease) receive evidence-based systematic care to reduce the risk of coronary event.

2   Ensure that all patients without established occlusive arterial disease who have a 30% risk of coronary even within 10 years receive evidence-based systematic care to reduce the risk of a coronary event. When this group of patients has been successfully managed, then treat all those whose 10-year risk of a coronary even is 15% or more.

3   Ensure the evidence-based prescription of ACE inhibitors, unless contraindicated, to all patients who may benefit. The patient groups are:
    a   Patients in (1) and (2)
    b   All diabetics

Building a heart failure register

1   Identify all patients with a diagnosis of heart failure on the practice register by:

- Searching the prescribing register for patients receiving a combination of loop diuretics and ACE inhibitors
- Opportunistically identifying patients attending for consultations who have a diagnosis of heart failure
- Searching for relevant Read-coded diagnoses on the computer, such as:

G58   Heart failure
G581-3   Left ventricular (LV) dysfunction
58531   Echocardiogram abnormal

2   Validate these lists by searching the medical records for a hospital diagnosis of heart failure, evidence of impaired LV function on echocardiogram or LV angiogram (performed during coronary arteriography), or evidence of heart failure on chest X-ray. Patients with evidence of supporting investigations or hospital diagnoses are termed 'confirmed heart failure' and those without, 'suspected heart failure'.

- Code suspected and confirmed heart failure cases with Read code G58 to enable the delivery of evidence-based systematic care to both groups

3   Ensure all new and previously diagnosed suspected cases of heart failure receive appropriate investigations (see Clinical Assessment).

Clinical assessment

- Breathlessness, fatigue and ankle swelling are the hallmark clinical symptoms of heart failure. Unfortunately, all three are very non-specific and are often found in other medical conditions

- Clinical assessment alone should not be used to diagnose heart failure as this can result in up to 50% inaccuracy of diagnosis

Referral for echocardiography

The referral process for echocardiography should be prioritized as follows:

- **1st priority** – all new suspected cases

- **2nd priority** – previously diagnosed suspected heart failure cases in the following order:
  - valvular heart disease
  - previous myocardial infarction (MI)
  - angina
  - atrial fibrillation

- **3rd priority** – those at highest risk of developing heart failure in the order of:
  - previous MI
  - clinical diagnosis of angina
  - diabetes
  - hypertension

Referral criteria

- In the first instance, this will be based on results of the following investigations:
  - baseline blood tests of FBC, U&Es, creatinine, LFT, TFT, RBS
  - resting 12-lead ECG
  - chest X-ray

- If results are **abnormal** – refer for echocardiography

- If the ECG is normal and the chest X-ray does not indicate cardiac pathology, then heart failure is virtually excluded and referral for echocardiography is unnecessary

- Persisting diagnostic uncertainty requires referral for a specialist opinion

Management following confirmation of diagnosis at the direct access echo service

Systolic heart failure confirmed

On results from hospital screening service:

- Review investigation

- Review management

- If LV dysfunction is confirmed, ensure that appropriate investigations are performed

and that evidence-based treatment is implemented

Non-drug therapy

Heart failure specific therapy

- Salt restriction
  - mild–moderate heart failure – restrict salt to 5–6 g/day
  - severe heart failure – restrict salt to 3–4.5 g/day

- Fluid restriction
  - avoid drinking large volumes over a short period, eg beer
  - severe heart failure – restrict daily volume to 1.5 litres when there are signs of fluid retention despite optimal therapy

- Patient and carer education
  - explain about the illness and the options for treatment to enable patients and their carers to participate in decision-making
  - enable self-management by explaining the benefits of symptom reporting and daily weighing (with reporting of a weight gain of 1.5 kg or more)
  - to improve compliance and reduce withdrawal from therapy, explain the benefits and effects of drug treatment
  - to prevent hospital admission/readmission
  - to develop support systems
  - suggest a progressive exercise programme for selected stable patients; walking or stationary cycling are suitable activities; activity may be limited by severity of heart failure, co-morbidities, or other health problems

Co-morbidity specific therapy

- Smoking cessation
- Weight reduction
- Regular exercise
- Diet

Drug therapy

- Start on a loop diuretic if patient is dyspnoeic and/or there are signs of fluid retention

- If heart failure is suspected, start an ACE inhibitor *at the same time* as a loop diuretic

- When starting an ACE inhibitor in a patient already taking a loop diuretic, stop the diuretic for 24 hours and give an initial small dose of ACE inhibitor (eg enalapril or lisinopril 2.5 mg, ramipril 1.25 mg) at bedtime to limit symptoms of hypotension. The next day, the dose is taken in the morning

- Titrate upwards the dose of ACE inhibitor at weekly increments (eg enalapril or lisinopril 5 mg) to the therapeutic maximum

- Monitor U&Es 3–4 days after each increment. Renal impairment may be seen at initial small doses and after dosage increments

- Stop up-titration if creatinine rises by >20% or increases to 180 μmol/l or more

- Prescribe an angiotensin II receptor blocker (ARB) if an ACE inhibitor is not tolerated due to an adverse reaction such as a rash or cough. It should be noted that both ARBs and ACE inhibitors can cause renal impairment

- Unless contraindicated, patients with NYHA class II or III who are stable and do not have excess fluid should be prescribed one of the recommended beta blockers

- Patients with respiratory disease can usually tolerate low dose cardioselective beta blockade. The starting dose is very low and, if tolerated, is increased by small amounts every two weeks to the target dose. Patients self-monitor and report symptom deterioration or a weight gain of 1.5 kg or more. About 10% of patients experience early worsening of heart failure:
  - mild worsening – temporarily increase diuretic
  - moderate worsening – increase diuretic and reduce beta blocker; after stabilization, increase beta blockers more slowly
  - dizziness and postural hypotension are relatively frequent and managed by staggering/changing doses of other hypotensive drugs

- Do not abruptly withdraw beta blockade. Reduce by 50% and taper off, if necessary

Drug	Starting dose	Target dose
Metoprolol SR	12.5–25 mg od	200 mg od
Bisoprolol	1.25 mg od	10 mg od
Carvedilol	3.125 mg od	25 mg bd

*Only carvedilol and bisoprolol are currently licensed for use in heart failure in the UK

- Patients with NYHA class III–IV or LV ejection fraction <35% who are receiving an optimum dose of ACE inhibitor or ARB will benefit from prescription of spironolactone 25 mg daily, but careful monitoring of U&Es is necessary

- Avoid prescription of NSAIDs as these counteract the effect of ACE inhibitors

- Review patients *quarterly*, when stable, with U&E check at each visit. Check medical treatment, BP, weight. Liaise with heart failure specialist nurse if NYHA class deterioration

- Avoid NSAIDs in patients with heart failure as these drugs antagonize the effects of ACE inhibitors and may interact with frusemide to cause interstitial nephritis

- Offer immunization against influenza/pneumonia

- Re-refer early for:
  - investigation and management of the cause of heart failure
  - management of co-morbidities
  - problems with symptom control or hypotension
  - acute decompensation
  - onset of significant intercurrent illness

Heart failure due to primary arrhythmia (usually AF)

- Treat atrial fibrillation (AF) with appropriate therapy

Heart failure due to valvular disease

- Refer to cardiology outpatient department unless already triggered by open access service

Normal echo

- Reconsider diagnosis especially regarding possible pulmonary aetiology

Appendix II: Hospital heart failure management guidelines

Hospital protocol for nonvalvular heart failure patients
Heart failure treatment pathway and protocol
Recommendations for hospital service

Establish both open access echocardiography service and open access heart failure services. The former provides echocardiography in conjunction with a medical opinion and the latter provides routine investigations if they have not already been carried out.

Open access echocardiography service requirements:

- Dedicated high quality echocardiography machine
- Dedicated senior echocardiographer
- Medical overview of reporting

Open access heart failure service requirements:
- Dedicated high quality echocardiography machine
- Dedicated senior echocardiographer
- Medical review of patient at each session
- Range of other investigations offered, ie:
  - ECG
  - chest X-ray (CXR)
  - routine laboratory investigations

Both services requirements:
- Medical records officer input
- Heart failure specialist nurse

Clinic input

- New patients with suspected heart failure

(direct GP referral with pre-referral ECG/CXR screening)

- Patients with a previous clinical diagnosis of heart failure (direct GP referral with pre-referral ECG/CXR screening)

- New acute admissions with suspected/clinical diagnosis of heart failure*

- *All* new admissions to coronary care unit (CCU) with a diagnosis of myocardial infarction (MI) or angina (unstable/acute/stable)*

- Referrals from consultants' outpatient clinics with a suspected or clinical diagnosis of heart failure

- Patients with high-risk conditions for heart failure (direct GP referral with ECG/CXR screening)

* Options for the identification of inpatients with heart failure or suspected heart failure:

- monitor admissions daily via heart failure service specialist nurse and/or heart failure service echocardiographer and/or bed manager for patients with a clinical diagnosis of heart failure on admission

  and/or

- liaise with pharmacy department for all inpatients being prescribed a *loop* diuretic

  and/or

- monitor discharge codes (for heart failure/MI/angina) – although this would be retrospective case identification and would delay diagnosis and initiation of appropriate therapy

Clinic operation

It is recommended that in order to maximize the medical cover available, open access echo services should run in parallel with consultant-led heart failure clinic services. The number of sessions required will depend on the predicted demand by the Trust and on the level of medical cover available.

- Daily
- First part of clinic for **CCU** echocardiograms

to identify new post MI and unstable angina patients with symptomatic and asymptomatic left ventricular (LV) dysfunction

- Second part of clinic for newly identified **inpatients** with suspected heart failure

- Third part of clinic for **open access** services

Estimated numbers

(based on 5% of admissions having heart failure and 10–12 echocardiograms possible each day)

Daily new inpatients with suspected heart failure	2–3
New MIs and inpatient angina patients	3–4
Open access referrals therefore available	3–4

Clinic output

GP open access referrals

- LV dysfunction confirmed – suggest appropriate ACE inhibitor/diuretic treatment and refer for follow-up in heart failure follow-up clinic and joint care with GP. However, if there is no heart failure follow-up clinic, refer back to GP or general cardiology clinics. Include patient education from heart failure specialist nurse at this visit. Liaison with primary care via heart failure specialist nurse

- Significant valvular disease – refer to general cardiology

- Primary atrial fibrillation (AF) – refer back to GP

- Noncardiac – refer back to GP

Inpatients (acute admissions, general and CCU)

- LV dysfunction confirmed – provide treatment recommendations regarding diuretics, ACE inhibitors, beta blockers

- Significant valvular disease – refer to cardiology

- Primary AF – standard treatment recommendations

- Noncardiac – further noncardiac investigations under general medicine

Hospital protocol for nonvalvular heart failure patients

For all patients:

- Bed rest

- Monitor daily weight aiming for weight loss of 1 kg per day (consider fluid balance chart in addition at least during acute/unstable phase)

- Restrict fluid to 1–1.5 litres per day

- Restrict salt intake (no added salt, avoid high salt content foods)

- Ensure all routine investigations complete, ie U&Es, FBC, TFTs, ECG, CXR

- Ensure on adequate loop diuretic, ie frusemide 40–120 mg daily. For acute heart failure switch to intravenous use. For chronic resistant heart failure, consider oral bumetanide instead of frusemide

- When stable and if U&Es are satisfactory, start ACE inhibitor:
  - enalapril 2.5 mg od
  - lisinopril 2.5 mg of
  - ramipril 1.25 mg of

- Check daily U&Es and if satisfactory up-titrate ACE inhibitor dosage. If creatinine increases >20% or reaches >180 µmol/l, reduce diuretic dose if possible, but if creatinine still >180 µmol/l, reduce ACE inhibitor dosage

- If ACE inhibitors are contraindicated or not tolerated then consider an angiotensin II receptor blocker (losartan or valsartan) or hydralazine + nitrates

- When stable and in NYHA class II–III heart

failure add a beta blocker (see table) and titrate up slowly according to data sheet

Drug	Starting dose	Target dose
Metoprolol SR	12.5–25 mg od	200 mg od
Bisoprolol	1.25 mg od	10 mg od
Carvedilol	3.125 mg od	25 mg bd

*Only carvedilol and bisoprolol are currently licensed for use in heart failure in the UK

If not stable after ACE inhibitor commencement and signs of fluid retention remain, do not start beta blocker but consider spironolactone 25 mg od and monitor K$^+$ daily. If signs of fluid retention remain and weight loss is inadequate, add metolazone 2.5 mg od and monitor U&Es daily, reducing the dose to alternate days when diuresis starts, then to twice weekly

- If concomitant AF, anticoagulate long term

- If associated high grade arrhythmias, add amiodarone and consider implantable defribrillator as per current guidelines

- Avoid NSAIDs as these offset the efficacy of ACE inhibitors

- Aim to discharge on maximum tolerated ACE dose, on appropriate loop diuretic dose and on beta blockade with appropriate lifestyle advice. On discharge, liaise with GP regarding further treatment and future monitoring. If appropriate, arrange follow-up in heart failure clinic/general cardiology outpatient department

- In patients with concomitant chest pain, oral/transdermal nitrates and/or amlodipine may be helpful and consider exercise testing (? revascularization possibilities) for diagnosis of aetiology and objective measure of exercise capacity

- Complete audit sheet

Heart failure treatment pathway and protocol

Admission

- Admit to designated ward if NYHA class II–III

- Consider admission to CCU if NYHA class IV or if arrhythmia (AF, ventricular tachycardia) responsible

- Admit to CCU if heart failure is due to recent/new MI

Refer to heart failure service

- Refer patient at earliest opportunity to heart failure service via ECG department for echocardiography

- CCU staff to telephone heart failure specialist nurse at 0845 each day with names of patients admitted in preceding 24 hours with a diagnosis of MI (Q wave or non-Q wave) or angina

- Admitting team to telephone heart failure specialist nurse at 0900 each day with names and location in hospital of patients admitted in preceding 24 hours with a presumptive diagnosis of heart failure

- Bed manager to telephone heart failure specialist nurse at 0915 each day with names and location in hospital of patients admitted in preceding 24 hours with a presumptive of heart failure

- Heart failure specialist nurse and heart failure echocardiographer to arrange echocardiography times for each patient (in the order of CCU patients first and general patients second)

Urgent echocardiogram

- All patients should have an echocardiogram **within** 24 hours of admission

Treatment protocol

Inpatient treatment recommendations for CCU patients

Follow inpatient protocol as above but note:

- If clinical/radiographic evidence of heart failure – commence ACE inhibitor when haemodynamically stable (BP >100 mmHg,

HR <100 bpm, urine output >600 ml in 24 hours, creatinine <170 µmol/l). This can precede but not replace the results of echocardiography

- If systolic dysfunction post MI – commence ACE inhibitor when haemodynamically stable (BP >100 mmHg, HR <100 bpm, urine output >600 ml in 24 hours, creatinine <170 µmol/l)

- If systolic dysfunction in angina – commence ACE inhibitor when haemodynamically stable (BP >100 mmHg, HR <100 bpm, urine output >600 ml in 24 hours, creatinine <170 µmol/l)

Note: ACE inhibitor therapy can precede – but in most patients will follow – beta blocker therapy in CCU patients

- Ensure all other investigations and treatment recommendations as in management protocol above are completed, including liaison with heart failure specialist nurse

Inpatient treatment recommendations for ward patients

Follow management protocol as above, but note:

- Refer to cardiology those patients where heart failure is secondary to acute/chronic valvular disease, suspected myocarditis or where patients have resistant heart failure or deteriorating heart failure despite medical treatment

- In patients with resistant heart failure – consider the addition of metolazone to loop diuretic, the use of inotropes, etc

- In patients with heart failure due to ischaemic heart disease – consider additional long acting nitrate therapy and/or amlodipine and aspirin

- Consider formal exercise testing when stable with view to revascularization

- In patients with heart failure and AF – consider oral anticoagulation and DC cardioversion

- Consider beta blocker therapy/amiodarone/implantable defibrillator for patients with symptomatic high-grade ventricular arrhythmias and impaired LV function

- When stabilized on medical treatment, refer to heart failure specialist nurse (via ECG department) for patient education – all patients should be seen prior to discharge

- Aim to discharge on maximum tolerated ACE inhibitor dose, on appropriate loop diuretic dose and on beta blockade with appropriate lifestyle advice. On discharge, liaise with GP regarding further treatment and future monitoring. If appropriate, arrange a follow-up in heart failure clinic/general cardiology outpatient department

- Complete heart failure audit sheet

Recommendations for hospital service

1 A dedicated echocardiography machine is available at each Trust

2 A dedicated senior echocardiographer is employed at each Trust

3 A specialist heart failure nurse is appointed for each Trust

4 A cardiologist with a specific interest in heart failure is identified in each Trust to lead the clinical service

5 The primary care service is open access echocardiography but with one or two sessions for open access heart failure clinics (providing clinical opinion and other investigations other than just echocardiography)

Index

Page numbers in *italics* refer to information that is shown only in a table or figure.